MAKING SENSE of
Fluids and Electrolytes

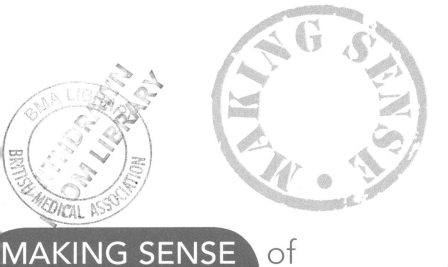

MAKING SENSE of
Fluids and Electrolytes

A hands-on guide

Zoja Milovanovic
Anaesthetic Clinical Fellow, Homerton Hospital
London, UK

Abisola Adeleye
Junior doctor training in Obstetrics and Gynaecology
in the East of England, UK

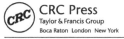
CRC Press
Taylor & Francis Group
Boca Raton London New York

CRC Press is an imprint of the
Taylor & Francis Group, an **informa** business

CRC Press
Taylor & Francis Group
6000 Broken Sound Parkway NW, Suite 300
Boca Raton, FL 33487-2742

© 2017 by Taylor & Francis Group, LLC
CRC Press is an imprint of Taylor & Francis Group, an Informa business

No claim to original U.S. Government works

Printed in Great Britain by Ashford Colour Press Ltd

International Standard Book Number-13: 978-1-4987-4719-6 (Paperback)

Visit the Taylor & Francis Web site at
http://www.taylorandfrancis.com

and the CRC Press Web site at
http://www.crcpress.com

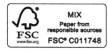

Contents

Acknowledgements

We have a number of people to thank for this book, without whom realisation of our idea would not have been possible. The Royal Society of Medicine for awarding us the young author's prize in 2013 and Dr Harpreet Gill for her collaboration in this.

Dr Douglas Corrigall, for his contribution to the design and content of the book, especially the medical chapter.

Our editorial advisors Dr Thomas Gilkes, Dr Stefanie Robert and Dr Shilpa Reddy for their clinical experience and for sharing our vision.

We are also deeply grateful to our families for their unwavering support and endurance during the writing of this book, and we would especially like to thank Mr Alex Hayes for his help and patience with proofreading our final copy.

List of abbreviations

A&E	accident and emergency
AAA	abdominal aortic aneurysm
ABG	arterial blood gas
ACE	angiotensin converting enzyme
ADH	antidiuretic hormone
AF	atrial fibrillation
AKI	acute kidney injury
ALP	alkaline phosphatase
ALS	advanced life support
ALT	alanine aminotransferase
APTT	activated partial thromboplastin time
AST	aspartate aminotransferase
ATP	adenosine triphosphate
AVPU	alert, responsive to voice, responsive to pain, unresponsive
AXR	abdominal x-ray
BE	base excess
BMI	body mass index
BNF	British National formulary
BNP	brain natriuretic peptide
BP	blood pressure
BSA	burn surface area
CCF	congestive cardiac failure
CK	creatinine kinase
CKD	chronic kidney disease
CMV	cytomegalovirus
COPD	chronic obstructive pulmonary disease
CPAP	continuous positive airway pressure
CRP	c-reactive protein
CRT	capillary refill time
CT	computed tomography
CVP	central venous pressure
CXR	chest x-ray
Da	daltons
DI	diabetes insipidus

DIC	disseminated intravascular coagulation
DKA	diabetic ketoacidosis
GCS	Glasgow Coma Scale
EBV	Epstein-Barr virus
ECF	extracellular fluid
ECG	electrocardiogram
ECHO	echocardiogram
EF	ejection fraction
eGFR	estimated glomerular filtration rate
ERCP	endoscopic retrograde cholangiopancreatography
FBC	full blood count
FFP	fresh frozen plasma
G&S	group and save
GI	gastrointestinal
GORD	gastro-oesophageal reflux disease
GP	general practitioner
GTN	glyceryl trinitrate
Hb	haemoglobin
HCl	hydrochloric acid
HDU	high dependency unit
HES	hydroxyethyl starch
HF	heart failure
HLA	human leucocyte antigen
HPA	human platelet antigen
HR	heart rate
HRS	hepatorenal syndrome
HTN	hypertension
ICF	intracellular fluid
ICU	intensive care unit
IHD	ischaemic heart disease
IM	intramuscular
INR	international normalised ratio
ITU	intensive therapy unit
IU	international units
IVF	intravenous fluids
JVP	jugular venous pressure
KDIGO	kidney disease improving global outcomes
HIV	human immunodeficiency virus
LFTs	liver function tests
LVEF	left ventricular ejection fraction
MAP	mean arterial pressure

MI	myocardial infarction
MONAC	morphine, oxygen, nitroglycerine, aspirin, clopidogrel
MRCP	magnetic retrograde cholangiopancreatography
MRI	magnetic resonance imaging
NBM	nil by mouth
NGT	nasogastric tube
NIV	non-invasive ventilation
NJT	nasojejunal tube
NICE	National Institute for Health and Clinical Excellence
NSAIDs	non-steroidal anti-inflammatory drugs
PCR	protein:creatinine ratio
PEA	pulseless electrical activity
PEG	percutaneous endoscopic gastrostomy
PMH	past/previous medical history
PND	paroxysmal nocturnal dyspnoea
PT	prothrombin time
RAS	reticular activating system
RAAS	renin-angiotensin-aldosterone system
RBC	red blood cell
RMP	resting membrane potential
RR	respiratory rate
SBP	systolic blood pressure
SBP	spontaneous bacterial peritonitis
SIADH	syndrome of inappropriate antidiuretic hormone secretion
SIRS	severe inflammatory response syndrome
SNS	sympathetic nervous system
SOB	shortness of breath
SSRIs	selective serotonin reuptake inhibitors
TCRE	transcervical resection of the endometrium
TEN	toxic epidermal necrolysis
TIPSS	transjugular intrahepatic portosystemic shunt
TRALI	transfusion-associated lung injury
TURP	transurethral resection of the prostate
U&Es	urea and electrolytes
USS	ultrasound scan
VBG	venous blood gas
VF	ventricular fibrillation
VT	ventricular tachycardia
vWF	von Willebrand factor
WBC	white blood cell count

How to use this book

This is a clinical companion to be used for the treatment of fluid balance, electrolyte and acid–base disorders. In the first chapter, fluid assessment and investigation will be reviewed. Subsequent chapters will implement this format as a quick reference for management of patients with various medical and surgical presentations. Each chapter will have the following layout:

Fluid assessment:
- History
- Examination
- Investigations

Management:
- Treat the underlying cause
- Treat the current fluid status
- Review of the implemented treatment

Special considerations:
- Guidelines and recommendations
- Subspecialties
- Electrolytes
- Acid–base

Fluid balance assessment is a crucial aspect of management of all patients on intravenous fluid (IVF) therapy and patients who have any signs or symptoms of fluid abnormality. The *National Institute for Clinical Excellence (NICE)* guidelines recommend daily review, including blood tests, of all patients on fluid therapy. Fluid balance assessment is the responsibility of the whole health care team. Fluid status abnormalities can be detected by nursing staff via patient symptoms and observations, by biochemistry and haematology lab scientists from blood test results and also during clinical examination by doctors, nurses and allied health care professionals.

This is not a recipe book on prescription of IVF; it is a tool to be used to guide your clinical judgement. Management should be tailored to an individual patient's fluid status and medical problem. The advice contained in this book is taken from clinical and physiological textbooks, *NICE* guidelines, and from the authors' personal experience and standard clinical practice.

CHAPTER 1

Fluid assessment

FLUID ASSESSMENT – FORMAT

Fluid management requires a full clinical assessment with a particular focus on the systems that affect the water content of the body: cardio-vascular, renal, endocrine and gastrointestinal.

In your clinical assessment, you should focus on the patient's overall wellbeing, as well as the fluid status in the different compartments. It is crucial to gauge which compartment has an excess or deficit of fluid, as excess in one compartment does not automatically mean excess in all compartments. For example, a patient with peripheral oedema might actually have an intravascular fluid deficit that can manifest itself clinically through hypotension and tachycardia. This book focuses on these clinically challenging situations.

HISTORY

Current medical problem
Why is the patient in hospital?

It is important to know why the patient was admitted to hospital. Evaluating the course of their treatment, plus any further medical problems, is equally important. For example, a patient might have been admitted with bowel obstruction, but has subsequently had a myocardial infarction; hence both of these would be the 'current medical problem' and would affect fluid therapy.

Current fluid status

Consider the patient's fluid intake and causes of extra fluid losses: do they balance out?

History is the first step in fluid assessment. What has the patient taken in versus what has been excreted? Patients can usually tell you how much they have eaten and drunk and also roughly how much urine they have passed. It is good practice to correlate this information with the fluid balance chart.

Intake

Has their medical/surgical condition stopped them from drinking enough water? If so, have they had enough replacement for their age and size? Always assess a patient's nutrition while they are in the hospital; this is the responsibility of all health care professionals. For example, surgical patients might be 'nil by mouth' (NBM) and therefore require maintenance fluid therapy, as well as replacement intravenous fluids (IVF). Assess the quantity of input from the following:

- Oral intake: All types of fluid
- IVF: Note types of fluids (crystalloids, colloids, blood products) and electrolyte composition
- Parenteral feeding: Note electrolyte composition
- Enteral feeding via a nasogastric tube (NGT), nasojejunal (NJ) tube or a percutaneous endoscopic gastrostomy (PEG) tube

Output

Assess all routes of output and insensible losses a patient might have. This includes assessing the quantity of:

- Previous/current diarrhoea, vomiting, urination and faeces.
- Catheters, drains, stoma outputs, NGTs, NJs, PEGs.
- Third-space losses, which are those where fluids shift to a 'new' compartment which is an extension of the extracellular fluid (ECF). This is sometimes seen in paralytic ileus, peritonitis and

conditions causing 'leaking' from capillaries, such as anaphy-laxis and sepsis.

- Insensible losses, which are those that cannot be accurately measured but can contribute significantly to a patient's fluid losses (Figure 1.1):

  - Respiratory tract: Fluid that evaporates from the respiratory tract increases with increased respiratory rate, 'mouth breathers' and also in ventilated patients.
  - Skin: Sweating and pyrexia will increase fluid loss.
  - Surgical evaporation: Evaporation from exposed surgical sites during the operation.

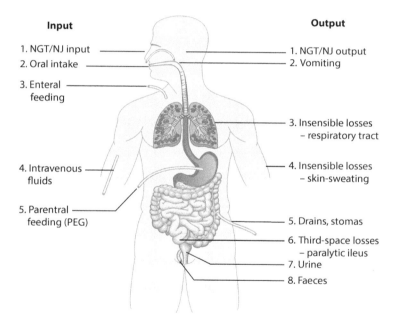

Input

1. NGT/NJ input
2. Oral intake
3. Enteral feeding
4. Intravenous fluids
5. Parentral feeding (PEG)

Output

1. NGT/NJ output
2. Vomiting
3. Insensible losses – respiratory tract
4. Insensible losses – skin-sweating
5. Drains, stomas
6. Third-space losses – paralytic ileus
7. Urine
8. Faeces

Figure 1.1   Diagram showing all input and output. (NGT, nasogastric tube; NJ, nasojejunal; PEG, percutaneous endoscopic gastrostomy.)

Signs and symptoms of fluid depletion/overload can be vague, but put in context with the fluid balance chart, they should support your diagnosis. It is important to look at trends as they will reveal the course of fluid abnormality. For example, a patient may become progressively hypotensive due to dehydration (if they are NBM with no replacement fluid given) and the observation chart will show a steady decline in blood pressure and a rise in heart rate.

Hypovolaemia

- **Symptoms:** thirst, oliguria/anuria, orthostatic hypotension, headache, lethargy, confusion, vomiting, diarrhoea
- **Signs:** decreased skin turgor, increased capillary refill time (>2 seconds), cool peripheries, dry mucous membranes, tachycardia, weak thready pulse, tachypnoea, hypotension, increased respiratory rate, coma

Hypervolaemia

- **Symptoms:** polyuria or oliguria, shortness of breath (SOB), orthopnoea
- **Signs:** peripheral and central oedema, ascites, raised jugular venous pressure (JVP), added heart sounds, basal crepitations on chest auscultation, increasing weight over a short period of time, headache, confusion, coma

Note: signs of hyponatremia might be present too (nausea, confusion, loss of appetite and general malaise).

Think about the different fluid compartments (Table 1.1).

Table 1.1   Signs and symptoms associated with each compartment

Compartment	Symptoms of hypovolaemia	Symptoms of hypervolaemia	Signs of hypovolaemia	Signs of hypervolaemia
Intravascular	Thirst, nausea		Tachycardia, hypotension	Raised JVP
Interstitial	Thirst, nausea	SOB, orthopnoea	No oedema, dry mucous membranes, poor skin turgor	Oedema, ascites In good hydration: moist mucous membranes, good skin turgor
Intracellular	Headache, coma		Difficult to assess directly	Difficult to assess directly

Past medical history

A patient's history will guide IVF prescribing. It should outline current fluid status and highlight any indications for cautious prescribing. Do they have a medical condition which will affect their body's ability to respond adequately to fluid deficiency or excess?

Focus on the following:

- **Cardiovascular:** Ischaemic heart disease (IHD) and heart failure (HF) will, in varying degrees, affect the heart's ability to pump blood around the body. Be cautious when prescribing fluid as decreased cardiac output might result in excess fluid outside the intravascular space, especially in patients with congestive cardiac failure (CCF). At the same time, it is important to aim for euvolaemia in these patients to ensure an adequate stroke volume and cardiac output (remember the Frank–Starling mechanism). Traditionally, getting the fluid balance right in this particular group of patients has always been a big challenge for doctors.

- **Renal:** Depending on the extent and cause of acute kidney injury (AKI) a patient may require extra fluids, or conversely they may require dialysis. Dehydration is one of the main causes of AKI, hence most patients require IVFs to manage their condition (a balanced crystalloid such as Hartmann's is generally the first choice). If, however, an AKI patient is oligo-anuric and develops clinical signs of fluid overload, in most cases this would be an indication for urgent renal replacement therapy. Chronic kidney disease (CKD) of varying degrees will affect how the body excretes fluids and electrolytes and hence the quantity and type of fluid required. Patients with end-stage renal failure may be on dialysis and no longer producing any urine; fluid therapy in these patients should be measured and conducted under senior guidance.

- **Hepatic:** Decompensated liver disease may affect sodium and water distribution so caution should be applied when prescribing fluids, especially sodium-containing fluids.

- **Gastrointestinal:** Excretion from the gastrointestinal tract can result in large fluid and electrolyte depletion (especially potassium and sodium), thus high stoma outputs, diarrhoea and vomiting all require regular electrolyte monitoring and aggressive fluid replacement.

- **Endocrine:** There are several endocrine conditions that can have a major impact on plasma osmolarity and, ultimately, the fluid composition of the body because of abnormalities in processing of sodium and glucose. Syndrome of inappropriate antidiuretic hormone secretion (SIADH) causes excess water retention which results in a lowered plasma osmolarity and low sodium. It can be caused by many conditions, including neurological and endocrine abnormalities, malignancy and infection, and can occur post-operatively. Deficiency of ADH (diabetes insipidus) will have the opposite effect, where too much water is secreted by the kidneys resulting in an increased plasma osmolarity. It can also be seen post-operatively, in malignancy or in head trauma. Uncontrolled diabetes mellitus also affects plasma osmolarity, as insufficient insulin results in increased plasma glucose that subsequently causes increased plasma osmolarity and draws water out of cells.

REMEMBER

Conservative fluid challenges and fluid therapy for patients with a history of: IHD, HF, CKD and on dialysis, decompensated liver disease.
Strict electrolyte management:
- *Potassium* in renal and heart disease
- *Sodium* in liver cirrhosis and HF

Medication

A thorough review of a patient's medication, including their drug history and current hospital drug chart, is essential. Some drugs will have a direct effect on electrolytes and fluid balance, as they act on the kidney and alter the composition of electrolytes excreted or retained. For example, loop diuretics increase the excretion of sodium and with this comes increased water excretion. Other drugs will affect the distribution of fluid by acting on the cardiovascular system or by attracting excess water into a compartment. For example, beta-blockers decrease heart rate and cardiac output. They can exacerbate acute cardiac failure and this can result in fluid seeping out of the vessels causing oedema.

Here, we review what impact drugs can have on patients' electrolytes and fluid requirements. For an up-to-date guide, please refer to the *British National Formulary (BNF)* or a clinical pharmacology textbook. Common drugs and their effect on fluid and electrolyte composition include the following:

- Calcium-channel blockers: Can cause ankle oedema.
- Angiotensin-converting enzyme (ACE) inhibitors: Can cause first dose hypotension and hyperkalaemia as well as sodium abnormalities.
- Beta-blockers: Can cause decreased cardiac output.
- Thiazide diuretics: Can cause hypokalaemia, hyponatraemia, oliguria, hyperglycaemia and hypercalcaemia.
- Loop diuretics: Can cause hypokalaemia, hyponatraemia, hyperglycaemia, hypocalcaemia, dehydration and hypovolaemia.
- Potassium-sparing diuretics: Can cause hyperkalaemia, hyponatraemia and water depletion.
- Some stimulant laxatives: Can cause dehydration and electrolyte imbalances.
- Electrolyte supplements: Increase the electrolyte in question. Potassium supplements will increase potassium, magnesium supplements will increase magnesium, etc.

EXAMINATION

Clinical assessment of patients relies on what can sometimes be very subtle signs. However, a constellation of signs in the context of a particular history should make the diagnosis easier and guide your investigations and management. Observations mainly provide an insight into the intravascular space, but when we are assessing patients it is important to address all three fluid compartments (Table 1.2 and Figure 1.2).

Table 1.2   Signs and symptoms that may occur in fluid balance disturbances

System	Fluid depletion	Fluid overload
Cardiovascular	• Tachycardia • Hypotension • Capillary refill time >2 seconds • Decreased skin turgor • Dry mucous membranes • Postural drop in blood pressure	• Hypertension • Added heart sounds • Raised JVP • Peripheral/sacral pitting oedema

(Continued)

Table 1.2 (*Continued*)   Signs and symptoms that may occur in fluid balance disturbances

System	Fluid depletion	Fluid overload
Respiratory	• Respiratory rate >20 breaths/min	• Oxygen saturation <92% • Respiratory rate >20 breaths/min • Bibasal crackles • Wheeze • Cyanosis
Renal	• Decreased urine output <0.5 mL/kg/hr • Concentrated urine	• Increased urine output >0.5 mL/kg/hr • Clear urine
Gastrointestinal	• Loose stool • High stoma output • Vomiting • Bowel obstruction	
Endocrine	• Blood sugar ≥11 mmol • Ketonuria	
Neurological	• Low Glasgow Coma Scale (GCS) <8 • Comatose	• Low GCS <8 • Comatose

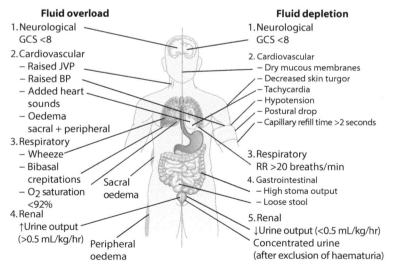

Fluid overload
1. Neurological
   GCS <8
2. Cardiovascular
   – Raised JVP
   – Raised BP
   – Added heart sounds
   – Oedema sacral + peripheral
3. Respiratory
   – Wheeze
   – Bibasal crepitations
   – O₂ saturation <92%
4. Renal
   ↑Urine output (>0.5 mL/kg/hr)

Sacral oedema

Peripheral oedema

Fluid depletion
1. Neurological
   GCS <8
2. Cardiovascular
   – Dry mucous membranes
   – Decreased skin turgor
   – Tachycardia
   – Hypotension
   – Postural drop
   – Capillary refill time >2 seconds
3. Respiratory
   RR >20 breaths/min
4. Gastrointestinal
   – High stoma output
   – Loose stool
5. Renal
   ↓Urine output (<0.5 mL/kg/hr)
   Concentrated urine
   (after exclusion of haematuria)

Figure 1.2   Diagram with clinical signs of fluid overload and fluid depletion. (BP, blood pressure; GCS, Glasgow Coma Scale; JVP, jugular venous pressure; RR, respiratory rate.)

INVESTIGATIONS

Blood tests

Blood tests should always be interpreted in the context of a patient's clinical state. Blood results provide an insight into what is happening to a patient and once again trends are crucial in letting you know whether the patient is essentially getting better or worse. For example, a patient might have a creatinine of 200 micromol/L, but the value itself is less helpful without the baseline and a clinical assessment of their fluid status (Table 1.3).

Table 1.3   Causes of electrolyte abnormalities

Electrolyte	Low level in . . .	High level in . . .

Sodium	SIADH
	Nephrotic syndrome
	Liver/cardiac/renal failure
	Diuretic excess
	Glucocorticoid deficiency
	Water overload, e.g. TURP
	  syndrome
		Diabetes insipidus
		Primary hyperaldosteronism
		Cushing's syndrome
		Excessive/incorrect normal
		  saline use (iatrogenic)

Potassium	Vomiting and/or diarrhoea Diuretic excess Pyloric stenosis Cushing's syndrome Renal tubular failure Conn's syndrome	Renal failure Potassium sparing diuretics Rhabdomyolysis Blood transfusion (large amount) Burns
Calcium	Acute pancreatitis Hypoparathyroidism Vitamin D deficiency Kidney disease	Hyperparathyroidism Malignancy Sarcoidosis
Phosphate	Re-feeding syndrome Hyperparathyroidism Diabetic ketoacidosis	Renal failure Rhabdomyolysis Malignancy
Magnesium	Malnutrition and malabsorption Chronic alcohol excess	Renal failure Hypothyroidism
Chloride	Vomiting	Hypernatremia Excessive normal saline use

Urea and electrolytes

Creatinine is generated by muscle breakdown and is produced at a constant rate in health. It is filtered out by the kidneys. It is a useful molecule to measure as it is released at a constant rate, thus changes in its concentration in the blood can be used to estimate the glomerular filtration rate. It is dependent on muscle mass and diet so patients with low or high muscle mass will have lower and higher baseline creatinine measurements. For example, an anorexic patient can have a low creatinine but still be in renal failure. For an average size person, a minimum of 400 mL of urine needs to be excreted per day to rid the body of these waste products.

Urea is a waste product of amino acid metabolism, secreted by the liver and filtered out by the kidneys. However, 40%–60% is actually reabsorbed in the medulla of the kidneys.

- Raised urea can be caused by sepsis and gastrointestinal bleeding (causing a high-protein load).
- Raised urea > raised creatinine (the so-called urea-to-creatinine ratio) can be caused by hypovolaemia leading to pre-renal failure.
- Raised urea along with raised creatinine can be caused by chronic kidney failure; the results should have been high for over a month.
- A low urea can be found in chronic liver disease.

REMEMBER

Common blood test results and their indications:

- FBC: Raised haemoglobin (Hb) and haemtocrit can occur in dehydration and conversely with aggressive fluid therapy. Raised white blood cells (WBCs) and platelets (and CRP) can be indicative of infection.
- U+E: Raised creatinine, urea and K^+ levels with AKI or CKD.
- Liver profile: Low albumin and raised clotting indicate hepatic dysfunction.
- Cardiac enzymes: Troponin, BNP.
- ABG: Base excess and lactate can be used as indicators of tissue perfusion (results must be interpreted in the clinical context).

Electrocardiogram

Essentials for assessment are the following:

- Any current cardiac ischemia or rhythm abnormality: Fluid therapy will depend on the extent and cause of the problem.

- Where possible look at previous electrocardiograms (ECGs) and compare for any signs of AF, ischaemia, MI new/old, conduction abnormality, dysrhythmias.
- Marked electrolyte abnormalities such as hypo/hyperkalaemia.

Imaging

Imaging can be useful to assess if there is abnormal fluid distribution fluid where it should not be, such as chest x-ray (CXR) findings in pulmonary oedema. Furthermore, imaging allows investigation into the clinical cause of abnormal fluid distribution, such as a cardiac or renal abnormality.

- X-ray: CXR for any signs of fluid overload.
- Echocardiogram: Left ventricular ejection fraction (LVEF), ventricular enlargement, right and/or left HF, distended or collapsed inferior vena cava.
- Ultrasound scan: Renal hydronephrosis, renal size, renal cysts/carcinoma.
- CT: CT of the abdomen for bowel obstruction and viscus perforation. CT of the chest for chronic pleural effusions and empyema.

A SYSTEMATIC APPROACH TO FLUID MANAGEMENT

This book aims to provide a systematic approach to IV fluid therapy as outlined in the following:

Treat the underlying cause

The basic management of common medical and surgical conditions will be briefly outlined. The main focus of this book is fluid management and as such this is not the source for specific in-depth medical and surgical management of the mentioned conditions. A senior's help should be sought whenever there is diagnostic uncertainty or when the patient is very unwell.

Treat the current fluid status

The specific fluid management for a particular condition will be recommended here but, of course, this must be tailored to your patient's other medical/surgical conditions, clinical examination and investigation findings.

Review of the implemented treatment

Any clinical intervention or treatment should be reviewed. Monitor the patient closely for any warning signs of fluid overload, dehydration, altered consciousness or other adverse outcomes. Ideally, an improvement in measured parameters should be seen following your treatment.

SPECIAL CONSIDERATIONS

- Guidelines: Relevant guidelines and scoring systems for the condition should be reviewed. The relevant aspects of the NICE guidelines on fluid therapy will be highlighted.
- Electrolytes: Specific considerations for electrolytes in each disease state. This should act as a reminder on how to manage electrolytes.

Further reading

Longmore M, Wilkinson IB, Davidson EH, Foulkes A and Mafi AR. *Oxford Handbook of Clinical Medicine*, 8th edition. Oxford, UK: Oxford University Press, 2010.

Olson J. *Clinical Pharmacology Made Ridiculously Simple*, 2nd edition. Miami, FL: Medmaster, 2003.

Smith K and Brain E. *Fluids and Electrolytes: A Conceptual Approach*, 2nd edition. Edinburgh, UK: Churchill Livingstone, 1991.

Chapter 2

Keeping the balance: physiology, electrolytes and intravenous fluids

INTRODUCTION

In this chapter, we review the physiology of fluid balance in the body. Electrolyte physiology, relevant investigations and management of electrolyte abnormalities are reviewed at the end of this chapter. To understand the fluid therapy we prescribe, it is necessary to know where the fluid goes, how it is distributed and what effects it has. To appreciate this, we need a good understanding of the different fluid compartments, how they are connected and what affects their composition (resulting in the clinical signs outlined in Chapter 1). To begin, we review the fluid composition of the human body. As this is a book about intravenous fluids (IVF), we also review currently used IVF, including their composition and most common uses. Water in the human body is intricately related to electrolytes and we cover the main electrolyte abnormalities, and their assessment, investigation and management. The end of this chapter contains a list of definitions of some essential concepts.

HUMAN BODY FLUID COMPARTMENTS

The human body consists roughly of two-thirds water, but this varies with age and total body percentage of adipose tissue. The usual values quoted are for an 'average' 70-kg man. In practice, however, the exact composition depends on several factors that have to be considered: gender, percentage of adipose tissue and age.

Most human cells consist largely of water, except adipose cells which are made up of 20% water. Women in general have more adipose tissue than men and this accounts for a decreased total percentage of body water in women: about 50% compared to 60% in men. Patients with more adipose tissue will contain less total body water when compared with individuals of the same size. However, size does have some bearing, and larger patients will obviously have a greater total amount of water than smaller patients. When considering obese patients it is useful to use ideal body weight as a starting point (in men, height in centimetres minus 100, and in women, height in centimetres minus 105), although other more complex and precise formulas exist.

As we age, the water content of our bodies decreases. Infants have a high proportion of total body water, approximately 70%, and this can increase with malnutrition (due to a relatively reduced amount of adipose tissue). The extra water is found in the interstitial space.

Water in the body is divided mainly into the intracellular fluid (ICF) compartment and extracellular fluid (ECF) compartment (see Figure 2.1). The ECF acts as a conduit between cells. Fluid can move slowly through the interstitium or quickly through plasma. As the fluid bathes the cells, it also affects their volume and osmolality, and the free passage of water ensures osmotic equilibrium.

In good health, water and electrolytes come from the intravascular compartment and are then redistributed across the whole body. Similarly, all the waste products made in the cells are ultimately excreted via plasma, the smallest compartment.

Water distribution: 2/3 inside the cells ICF (40% body weight)

1/3 outside the cells ECF (20% body weight)

1/4 of ECF is intravascular (5% body weight)

3/4 of ECF is interstitial (15% body weight)

It is worth remembering that there is also variation in electrolyte composition within cells. For example, the calcium gradient between the sarcoplasmic reticulum and cytoplasm in muscle cells is used to stimulate contraction. Electrolytes and associated clinical abnormalities are covered at the end of this chapter.

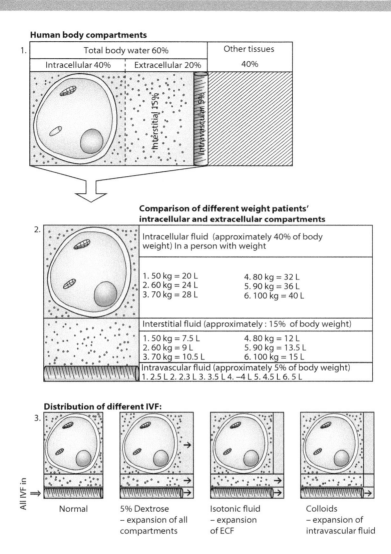

Figure 2.1 Diagram showing the different fluid compartments. The arrows indicate compartment expansion.

Fluid intake and output

Although there can be a massive variation in the amount of water and electrolytes ingested and excreted each day, it is useful to know some average figures so that you can estimate excess input/loss in patients (Table 2.1).

Table 2.1   Average water intake and output for an adult

Intake approximations (mL)	Output approximations (mL)
Oral fluids: 1500	Urine: 1500
Water released from food: 750	Faeces: 100
Metabolism: 250	Insensible losses: Skin perspiration: 500 Lungs (expired air): 400
Disease: IVF and medication, and abnormal oral intake	Disease: sweating, any other fluid
TOTAL 2500 mL approximation	TOTAL 2500 mL approximation

The actual composition of fluid is maintained very tightly by the body. Ion concentrations are essential for basic cell functions, such as action potentials and release of neurotransmitters. Although there might be massive variations in water and electrolyte intake, ion composition and osmolality are maintained within very tight limits. Abnormalities can occur when patients are not able to ingest an adequate amounts of water and electrolytes (for example when they are unconscious or nil by mouth [NBM]) or when there is a problem with filtering of plasma, such as in kidney disease.

Essential intake of water and electrolytes is achieved through eating and drinking. *National Institute for Health and Care Excellence* guidelines (NICE Guideline 2013) outline the basic daily requirement of water, glucose and electrolytes. Sometimes, IVF is the only viable source of these basic requirements, for example when the patient is NBM prior to surgery.

Table 2.2   Table of daily requirements

Substance	Daily requirement
Water	25–30 mL/kg
Glucose	50–100 g
Sodium/potassium/chloride	1 mmol/kg

Source: NICE Guideline. *Intravenous Fluid Therapy in Adults in Hospital.* 2013. https://www.nice.org.uk/guidance/cg174.

The values in Table 2.2 are only the basic requirements and additional losses must be added on, for example excess water, potassium and chloride are lost in patients who are vomiting.

So a fluid regime of '1 salty and 2 sweet' (1 L of 0.9% saline and 2 L of 5% dextrose) would provide the following:

- 3 L of water: Required maintenance amount for 100-kg man
- 100 g of glucose: Required amount
- 150 mmol of sodium: Required maintenance amount for 150-kg man
- 150 mmol of chloride: Required maintenance amount for 150-kg man
- 0 mmol of potassium: Deficit of 70 mmol for 70-kg man

This regime has been used in the past, with addition of potassium to IVF, so as to avoid hypokalaemia.

So, it is clear that one should tailor fluid therapy to individual patients and not prescribe the same for all, even on busy night shifts! IVF is a prescription for a reason, the same as medication; it is not harmless and should only be prescribed when necessary.

Movement between the fluid compartments

There is constant movement of water and electrolytes between the compartments. The composition of each compartment is reliant on both the water and electrolyte content of the neighbouring compartment and the membrane that separates them. These factors determine the movement of water and ions.

1. **Cell membrane**

   There are divisions between all the fluid compartments, the most notable being between the ECF and ICF. The cell membrane supports these two different fluid compartments. There are differences in ion distribution between the ECF and ICF.

   a. **Cations:** SODIUM (Na^+) is the main ECF cation, POTASSIUM (K^+) is the main ICF cation.

   b. **Anions:** BICARBONATE (HCO_3^-) and CHLORIDE (Cl^-) are the main ECF anions, PROTEINS and PHOSPHATES (PO_4^-) are the main ICF anions.

   The gradients of ions and the charge across cell membranes are again tightly controlled in health. For example, the sodium–potassium-ATPase pump maintains the sodium and potassium gradients across the membrane. All movement of ions across membranes occurs through ion channels that can be active (requiring energy and working against the concentration gradient) or passive (down the concentration gradient). The interplay of these complex and fascinating processes is beyond the scope of this book. However, it is important to appreciate that maintenance of these gradients is crucial for proper cell-to-cell signalling and function of the various intracellular compartments. The composition of the fluid in the extracellular compartments is essential for this as it contributes to intracellular water and ion composition.

Despite the differences in ion composition, ICF and ECF will have the same osmolality in health, generally (within the range of 275–295 mOsm/kg apart from in the Loop of Henle in the kidney). If there is increased osmolality in the ECF, it will affect the ICF osmolality. An osmotic gradient will be created and water will be distributed down the gradient until it is spread equally.

2. **Capillary wall**

The capillary wall divides the intravascular compartment (plasma) and the interstitium. However, there is constant movement of water and electrolytes between the two compartments due to large proteins being higher in concentration in the plasma and being unable to move across the capillary membrane. These large proteins will exert an oncotic effect which is counteracted by hydrostatic pressure created by contraction of the arterial wall. This moves water out of the arteries. The hydrostatic pressure decreases down the vascular tree, and in the veins it is less than the oncotic pressure (which is constant throughout).

Osmotic gradients, due to plasma proteins creating an oncotic pressure, draw fluid into the plasma from the surrounding tissue. Hydrostatic forces in the arteries push fluid into the interstitium from the plasma. Thus, there is a continuous movement of fluid between plasma and interstitium.

Starling's hypothesis states that there is continuous filtration of fluid across the semi-permeable membrane due to the oncotic and hydrostatic forces. Movement of fluid out of the intravascular compartment is due to higher hydrostatic pressure compared to oncotic pressure in the arteries (pushing fluid out). Movement of fluid into the intravascular compartment is due to higher oncotic pressure compared to hydrostatic pressure in the veins (pulling fluid in). Both of these forces should ultimately balance out and if they do not this can result in oedema.

Starling's Equation

Net filtration pressure = (C *hydrostatic* – I *hydrostatic*) – (C *oncotic* – I *oncotic*)

C – Capillary	*hydrostatic* – Hydrostatic pressure
I – Interstitial	*oncotic* – Oncotic pressure

RENAL PHYSIOLOGY

Kidneys filter plasma volume, electrolytes and remove waste products. The kidneys also maintain a normal pH and have an endocrine function; they regulate red blood cell volume via erythropoietin, and calcium levels in the blood via parathyroid hormone and vitamin D metabolism.

The nephron

Kidneys regulate plasma composition via the nephron, by filtering plasma.

- **Glomerulus and Bowman's capsule.** Plasma is filtered from the glomerulus into Bowman's capsule at a rate of 125 mL/min. The constriction of the afferent and the dilatation of the efferent arterioles cause a high hydrostatic pressure of 45 mmHg. Small particles are forced through into Bowman's capsule whilst larger proteins remain behind due to their size.

- **Proximal tubule.** Most reabsorption occurs here. Seventy percent of the ultrafiltrate (particles and water minus any large particles) is returned back to plasma.

  - Most of the filtered *sodium* is reabsorbed here, pulling *water* back into the vessels with it.

  - *Glucose* and *amino acids* are completely reabsorbed here, using sodium as a passive co-transporter.

  - *Potassium* is also mostly reabsorbed here; against its gradient and presumably in exchange with H^+ ions.

- H^+ *ions* are mostly excreted here; however, the pH of the solution only drops by 0.4 (from 7.4 to 7) because the HCO_3^- is mainly (90%) reabsorbed here thus acting as a buffer.
- *Urea* is concentrated here but due to the high gradient thus created, it is reabsorbed back into plasma.
- *Calcium and phosphate* are passively reabsorbed here.

- **Loop of Henle.** This part of the nephron concentrates the urine. It does this by creating a large osmotic gradient in the medulla so that water is drawn out of the ultrafiltrate back into the capillary bed.

  Renal medulla osmolality is between 900 and 1400 mOsm/kg (much higher than the 285 mOsm/kg in the plasma) and is created by active transportation of chloride, which is followed by sodium, into the medulla from the thick ascending limb. Urea contributes to the medullar osmolality as it leaves the distal collecting tubule down its gradient (once it becomes permeable to urea in the medulla) where it is concentrated. The descending limb of the loop is the only area in the whole loop permeable to water and this is where water leaves the ultrafiltrate (although most of it is reabsorbed in the proximal tubule). This is the **countercurrent exchange system** helped by vessels that follow the course of the loop (vasa recta); sodium chloride is excreted in the ascending limb (which becomes hypo-osmotic at 100 mOsm/kg) and it causes water to be reabsorbed in the descending limb due to the surrounding high medullar osmolality. *Magnesium* is mostly reabsorbed here.

- **Distal and collecting tubules.** These absorb only 5% of the filtered electrolytes but control the final composition of the urine via the actions of aldosterone and antidiuretic hormone (ADH). Ultrafiltrate coming into the distal tubule has a low osmolality which drops further (from 100 to 50–75 mOsm/kg) because of their impermeability to water. Sodium is reabsorbed in the collecting duct and potassium is secreted due to aldosterone.

Hormones

- **Aldosterone.** Reabsorbs sodium via three mechanisms in the collecting ducts: it increases membrane permeability to sodium, Na^+ exchange for H^+ both on the tubular surface and at the Na^+/K^+ pump on the capillary surface. Similarly, aldosterone increases permeability to K^+ which actually moves down its gradient from the cells into the tubule passively. High potassium levels will cause the secretion of aldosterone from the adrenal cortex. It also increases sodium reabsorption from sweat and tears.

- **ADH.** Also known as vasopressin, ADH acts on the distal tubule and collecting ducts to increase permeability to water via water channels. Thus, water is reabsorbed back into the capillary down its gradient due to the hypertonicity of the surrounding medulla. It is activated by osmoreceptors in the hypothalamus when sodium concentration increases, and by stretch receptors (baroreceptors) in the left atrium and large vessels when blood pressure decreases. (Figure 2.2).

REMEMBER

Glomerulus and Bowman's capsule: filter plasma particles and fluid out of the blood vessels.
Proximal tubule: reabsorption of most electrolytes, water, glucose and amino acids.
Loop of Henle: concentrates the urine by reabsorbing most of the water back down the osmolar gradient created by the countercurrent system.
Distal and collecting tubule: fine-tuning of the final urine electrolyte composition occurs here, and hence the regulation of pH and electrolyte composition of the blood. Aldosterone acts on the collecting duct to reabsorb sodium and ADH contributes to water reabsorption.

Renal handling of electrolytes

Sodium regulation is achieved via the following three main systems:

1. Renin–angiotensin–aldosterone system: sodium retention
2. Sympathetic nervous system: sodium retention
3. Atrial natriuretic factors: sodium excretion

Potassium is mainly reabsorbed in the proximal tubule and excreted in the collecting duct by aldosterone. Potassium exchange can affect the plasma pH.

Water is reabsorbed all along the nephron. The body content of water is regulated by the ADH and the thirst mechanism.

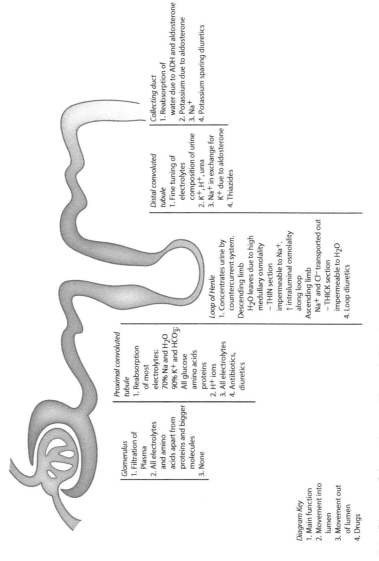

Glomerulus
1. Filtration of Plasma
2. All electrolytes and amino acids apart from proteins and bigger molecules
3. None

Proximal convoluted tubule
1. Reabsorption of most electrolytes: 70% Na and H_2O 90% K^+ and HCO_3^-; All glucose amino acids proteins
2. H^+ ions
3. All electrolytes
4. Antibiotics, diuretics

Loop of Henle
1. Concentrates urine by countercurrent system. Descending limb H_2O leaves due to high medullary osmolality
   – THIN section impermeable to Na^+.
   ↑ intraluminal osmolality along loop
   Ascending limb Na^+ and Cl^- transported out
   – THICK section impermeable to H_2O
4. Loop diuretics

Distal convoluted tubule
1. Fine tuning of electrolytes composition of urine
2. K^+, H^+, urea
3. Na^+ in exchange for K^+ due to aldosterone
4. Thiazides

Collecting duct
1. Reabsorption of water due to ADH and aldosterone
2. Potassium due to aldosterone
3. Na^+
4. Potassium sparing diuretics

Diagram Key
1. Main function
2. Movement into lumen
3. Movement out of lumen
4. Drugs

Figure 2.2   Diagram of the nephron and its main functions.

Sodium and water balance

The amount of water in the body is essentially determined by the amount of sodium. This is because water can freely move between all compartments and its osmosis is determined by the main ECF ion sodium.

Sodium plasma concentration reflects plasma osmolality in most cases, except when there are other solutes adding to the osmolality, such as glucose in diabetic ketoacidosis (DKA). Since the intake of water can vary dramatically, it has a great effect on osmolality. ADH and the thirst mechanisms are the main reasons plasma osmolality is maintained tightly between 275 and 295 mOsm/kg.

REMEMBER

Sodium status determines ECF volume. Decreased sodium in the ECF results in decreased ECF volume, and an increase in sodium in the ECF results in increased ECF volume.

Water status determines serum sodium concentration. Thus, serum sodium concentration is not the total amount of body sodium but the sodium concentration in ECF volume, i.e. the amount of water relative to the amount of sodium.

INTRAVENOUS FLUIDS

Introduction

Intravenous fluids (IVF) available for clinical practice include crystalloids, colloids and blood products (which will be covered in Chapter 6). Their clinical properties are unsurprisingly based on their constituents, electrolytes and molecules added, which in turn will have an effect on their surroundings once added to the human body. This property of IVF is called their tonicity (see definitions listed at the end of this chapter) and they can be further classified as isotonic, hypotonic or hypertonic. Tonicity is the attraction of water into a compartment based on its relative concentration of effective osmoles. In the human body, the compartment we are most concerned with are the cells, so tonicity is regarded in relation to water movement into and out of cells. Just a quick note on water first.

Water

Water comprises more than half of the human body and covers the majority of the planet, but it is a fluid we NEVER administer to patients (at least not intravenously!). In clinical practice, water is used for mixing some medication but it is never administered in pure form directly into the patient's vein. This is because water is hypotonic; the danger is that water can enter the cells in an unrestrained manner which can result in cell haemolysis. However, we will quickly review some properties of water as they affect the IVF we give to patients and also more widely influence how drugs work in the body.

Water has several special properties due to its covalent bonding and subsequent hydrogen bonds. These give it much higher melting and boiling points and a higher surface tension compared to similar molecules. Water is made of one oxygen atom sharing an electron with each of the two hydrogen atoms attached. Oxygen is a larger atom and attracts the shared electrons more than the hydrogen atoms, thus creating a polarity to these covalent bonds. The oxygen atom will have a slightly negative charge and the hydrogen a slightly positive one, resulting in an attraction between molecules called hydrogen bonds. Water is a polar solvent and so polar (hydrophilic) molecules will dissolve readily whereas non-polar (lipophilic) molecules will not; essentially similar molecules will dissolve each other. The slight negative and positive charge on the oxygen and hydrogen atoms help water dissolve ionic molecules by surrounding them and attracting oppositely charged ions. This means that water is a very good solvent in which ionic metals and non-metals can be dissolved, such as sodium, chloride, potassium and calcium.

Colloids

Colloids are IVFs used to expand intravascular volume, as they are meant to act using the same way as endogenous proteins and increase the intravascular oncotic pressure. This increased oncotic pressure is hypothesised to retain the fluid in the intravascular space for longer and attract water into the intravascular space. In theory, colloids provide much more fluid in the intravascular space (nearly all of the colloid given), in comparison with a much smaller percentage of crystalloid (depending on its tonicity) which is also distributed to other compartments. There has been a longstanding debate on the use of colloids versus crystalloids for resuscitation of unwell patients. Colloids are more expensive and occasionally can cause serious side effects such as exacerbation of acute kidney injury and coagulopathies. Some colloids have also been linked with anaphylaxis. There has been a meta-analysis of the use of colloids versus crystalloids in resuscitation, which showed no benefit of starches, a subgroup of high-molecular colloids. Some of the starches, for example hydroxyethyl starch (HES), have actually been withdrawn from clinical use because their serious side effects do not outweigh their benefits. This is not a forum for review of the latest research but there have been some significant studies regarding the use of colloids; please see the references in the 'Further Reading' section.

The term colloid describes a mixture of two or more substances that are evenly mixed; this can include gases, liquids or solids mixed in a solution. In clinical practice, these fluids include particles greater than 10,000 Da and it is these larger molecules that allow the solution to exert oncotic pressure and maintain water in the intravascular compartment. The larger molecules are either from animal, plant or glucose base; we will review each type of colloid in turn.

1. **Gelatins**

   Gelatins are semi-synthetic colloids made from animal connective tissue (hydrolysed collagens). The protein molecules are 30,000 Da and cannot cross the capillary membrane so will remain in the plasma, but side effects can include anaphylaxis. Patients should be asked (where practical) prior to their use, as some may object on a religious basis.

   An example is *Gelaspan* which is composed of modified gelatin, a succinylated gelatin with molecular weight of 26,500 Da.

   Content of Gelaspan: Na^+ 151 mmol/L, K^+ 4 mmol/L, Cl^- 103 mmol/L, Ca^{2+} 1 mmol/L, Acetate 24 mmol/L, Mg^{2+} 1 mmol/L, and 40 g of succinylated gelatin in 1000 mL.

2. **Starches**

   Starches are made from plant extracts, amylopectins linked with a hydroxyethyl group. These colloids can persist in the circulation up to 24 hours after administration due to their large molecular size (they have a wide range of molecular size up to 200,000 Da). They are expensive to produce. An example is HES 10%.

   Starches can lead to the following side effects: persistent itch, coagulopathy, exacerbation of acute kidney injury and risk of anaphylaxis (smaller than gelatins). Their serious side effects have resulted in their removal from use in the United Kingdom (Government Medical Safety Alert for HES 2013).

3. **Dextrans**

   Dextrans are made from glucose polymers. For example, Dextran 70 has molecules of 70,000 Da in weight. It increases oncotic pressure but also decreases plasma viscosity. It can cause hyperglycaemia and hyperosmolality, as it also contains sodium chloride and is a hyperosmolar IVF.

4. **Albumin**

   Albumin is a naturally occurring protein and is developed from human albumin. It comes in varying strengths (5% and 20% albumin in 0.9% saline), and is isotonic in the lower concentrations of up to 5%. It is commonly used as the IVF of choice during ascitic drainage to avoid large fluid shifts. It can cause hypersensitivity reactions.

Summary

Several points for thought regarding colloid use:

- Colloids should be used for resuscitation only and not maintenance.
- Colloids are of value in hypovolemic resuscitation, but in haemorrhagic shock, replace blood with blood (Chapter 6).
- Colloids are usually diluted in a 0.9% saline-type solution and their use can result in variable results.
- Use of certain colloids can result in renal injury and anaphylaxis.
- Gelatins are the most commonly used synthetic colloids.

In conclusion, the evidence supporting the use of colloids over crystalloids for resuscitation remains equivocal (see Chapter 3). There is no evidence to support the use of starch-containing solutions and some evidence that they may be harmful; they should not be used and are described here for the sake of completeness.

Individual clinical practice will vary regarding the use of colloids over crystalloids in certain situations such as resuscitation in a cardiac arrest. It is, however, worth noting that the use of balanced crystalloids, such as Hartmann's or Plasmalyte, is recommended by national and international guidelines for administration in the unwell adult patient (e.g. *NICE, KDIGO, Surviving Sepsis Campaign*).

Crystalloids

Crystalloids consist of water with the addition of ions and/or glucose in differing proportions. Composition of ions and glucose will have an effect on the distribution of the IVF through the body's fluid compartments, depending on whether they are isotonic, hypertonic or hypotonic as compared to plasma.

Isotonic fluids

Isotonic fluids aim to have a very similar osmolarity to plasma by roughly mimicking its cation and anion composition, especially with regard to plasma's effective osmoles. Since these fluids contain ions in an isotonic composition, i.e. they aim to be the same as plasma, they will theoretically distribute evenly through the whole of the ECF. The solutes are small molecules and they will pass freely across the capillary semi-permeable membrane but they will not be able to freely enter the cell because of the cell lipid bilayer membrane. Hence, isotonic crystalloids will not directly affect the composition of the cell like hypotonic fluids; they will not provide water that can enter directly into the cells. These fluids essentially have effective osmoles which will retain water within its compartment, the ECF.

Isotonic crystalloids distribute evenly through ECF; approximately only 25% will remain in the intravascular space and 75% will be in the interstitial space. This means that out of 1 L of crystalloid only 250 mL will remain in blood. Due to their tonicity, larger volumes of isotonic crystalloids, compared to colloids or blood, are needed for intravascular expansion. Due to ECF distribution, excessive use of any IVF can result in peripheral oedema and an increase in intravascular pressure. Depending on the patient and their current physiology, especially cardiac function, this may put strain on their heart and result in pulmonary oedema. In cases of sepsis, the capillary membranes become 'leaky' (see Chapter 3 for more on this) due to the action of proinflammatory cytokines. The key is, as always, to carefully monitor your patient and their response.

0.9% normal saline

Content: Na^+ 154 mmol/L, K^+ 0 mmol/L, Cl^- 154 mmol/L, Osmolarity 308 mOsm/L.

The chloride content is higher than in plasma (95–105) and therefore, excess use can result in a hyperchloraemic acidosis. Over the past few years, more evidence has emerged indicating that hyperchloraemic states can result in worse patient outcomes. Hyperchloraemia appears to impair splanchnic and renal blood flow and interfere with T-cell function and the coagulation system. Hence, most national guidelines – for example *NICE, Kidney Disease: Improving Global Outcomes (KDIGO), Acute Kidney Injury (AKI), Surviving Sepsis Campaign* – are now endorsing the use of balanced crystalloids, such as Hartmann's or Plasmalyte, for resuscitation. However, it is one of the most widely available and used crystalloids on medical and surgical wards. One advantage of normal saline is that we can supplement potassium.

Sodium and the resulting osmolarity are also slightly higher than in plasma and, with excess use, can result in more sodium in the ECF and hence water, resulting in increased volume (peripheral oedema). Note that there is no potassium and use of this crystalloid alone could result in dangerous hypokalaemia. This can be countered by adding potassium to the fluid, usually in quantities of 20 or 40 mmol in 1 L (administration of potassium has to be done at a slow rate, see the electrolyte section in this chapter).

Physiologically balanced solutions

Crystalloids with an electrolyte composition similar to plasma are called physiologically balanced solutions and they are thought to be less physiologically disruptive than normal saline when used in large quantities, as they should not produce an acidosis.

1. **Ringers**

   Content: Na^+ 147 mmol/L, K^+ 4 mmol/L, Cl^- 156 mmol/L, Ca^{2+} 2.2 mmol/L, Osmolarity 309 mOsm/L.

   Sodium and potassium are within plasma range.

2. **Hartmann's (Lactated Ringer's solution)**

   Content: Na^+ 131 mmol/L, K^+ 5 mmol/L, Cl^- 111 mmol/L, Ca^{2+} 2 mmol/L, Lactate (HCO_3^-) 29 mmol/L, Osmolarity 279 mOsm/L.

   Sodium, potassium and osmolarity are within plasma range, while chloride is marginally high. The human liver converts the sodium lactate component swiftly into bicarbonate and water. Hence, Hartmann's is an alkalising fluid which would be the ideal choice for patients with metabolic acidosis.

   Metabolic acidotic states often coincide with hyperkalaemia, as the body attempts to move H^+ ions out of the plasma and into the cell, which happens in exchange for potassium. However, if an alkalising fluid such as Hartmann's is administered, this process is reversed and the potassium moves back into the cell. By correcting the metabolic acidosis, the hyperkalaemia is addressed and corrected at the same time. The bicarbonate content quoted comes from the lactate molecule which uses H^+ ions and leaves the HCO_3^- instead.

3. **Plasmalyte 148**

   Content: Na^+ 140 mmol/L, K^+ 5 mmol/L, Cl^- 98 mmol/L, Gluconate 23 mmol/L, Acetate 27 mmol/L, Mg^{2+} 1.5 mmol/L, Osmolarity 295 mOsm/L.

   Isotonic fluid that also has an alkalising effect.

4. **1.26% Bicarbonate**

   Content: Na^+ 150 mmol/L, K^+ 0 mmol/L, Cl^- 0 mmol/L, Ca^{2+} 0 mmol/L, Bicarbonate (HCO_3^-) 150 mmol/L, Glucose 0 g, Osmolarity 300 mOsm/L (approximately, it is isotonic).

   Bicarbonate should be used under senior direction only. It can be used to replace bicarbonate in patients with low levels (<20 mmol/L) in a high dependency unit (HDU), for example in the context of acute kidney injury, which is a bicarbonate-losing state.

Hypotonic fluids

Hypotonic solutions have lower osmolarity and attract water less than the ICF. Essentially, they provide water to the cells by having a lower number of effective osmoles than the ICF and, therefore, water will go down its gradient into the cells and cause cell swelling. Hypotonic fluids will distribute evenly across all compartments, so 33% will remain in ECF (and of this only 25% in the intravascular compartment) and 66% will enter the cells. Their clinical use is fairly limited.

1. **5% Dextrose**

   Content: Glucose 50 g (50 mg/mL), Na^+ 0 mmol/L, K^+ 0 mmol/L, Cl^- 0 mmol/L, Ca^{2+} 0 mmol/L, Osmolarity 278 mOsm/L.

   Glucose is the only molecule besides water in this crystalloid and it is not an effective osmole in health (see earlier text). Once administered, glucose is taken up intracellularly by insulin and only water is left behind. Therefore, 1 L of 5% dextrose is equivalent to 1 L of water being administered (without the risk of haemolysis). It is a fluid that will hydrate the cells, but inversely it can cause hyponatremia if used in excess. It is not suitable for resuscitation, as much larger volumes would be needed, and only a small amount would remain in the intravascular space. This fluid should never be given to a hyponatraemic patient.

2. **0.45% Saline**

Content: Na^+ 75 mmol/L, K^+ 0 mmol/L, Cl^- 75 mmol/L, Ca^{2+} 0 mmol/L, Glucose 0 mmol/L, Osmolarity 150 mOsm/L.

This is half-strength saline that is used with caution in HDU settings to treat hypernatremia. Sodium levels must be checked regularly to ensure they are corrected slowly, generally not exceeding 0.5–1 mmol/L/hr.

3. **Dextrose/saline (0.18% saline + 4% dextrose)**

Content: Na^+ 30 mmol/L, K^+ 0 mmol/L, Cl^- 30 mmol/L, Ca^{2+} 0 mmol/L, Glucose 40 g, Osmolarity 284 mOsm/L.

Hypotonic fluid providing glucose and lower sodium content than 0.9% saline.

It should not be used as a maintenance fluid or in children under 16.

REMEMBER

Both dextrose and half-strength saline are used to treat hypernatremic states, but close monitoring in an HDU setting is required to ensure that the sodium levels normalise slowly (maximum 0.5–1 mmol/hr).

Hypertonic fluids

Hypertonic fluids have higher tonicity than plasma and cells, by having a higher concentration of effective osmoles compared to those found inside the cells. Administration of these fluids will result in a higher gradient of water outside the cell and water will move down its gradient out of the cells, essentially causing cell shrinkage. Since they can cause drastic changes in cell volume, they should be used under expert guidance only. An example would be 1.8%, 3%, 5% or 7.5% saline.

These hypertonic fluids are occasionally used in patients who have a traumatic brain injury and evidence of cerebral oedema, or in severely hyponatraemic patients who have had a seizure, or in cardiac arrest.

They should not be used outside the intensive therapy unit (ITU) unless under the care of a specialist team such as endocrinologists or in a neurosurgery unit (Table 2.3).

Table 2.3 Summary of commonly used crystalloids and their electrolyte composition

IVF	Sodium mmol/L	Potassium mmol/L	Chloride mmol/L	Glucose	Osmolarity mOsm/L	Additional
0.9% Normal saline	154	0	154	0	308	pH 5.5
Hartmann's	131	5	111	0	279	pH 6.5 Lactate 29 mmol/L Calcium 2 mmol/L
Plasmalyte 148	140	5	98	0	295	pH 6.5–8, Mg^{2+} 1.5 mmol/L Acetate 27 mmol/L Gluconate 23 mmol/L
Dextrose/ saline (0.18% saline + 4% dextrose)	30	0	30	40 g	284	
5% Dextrose	0	0	0	50 g	278	
0.45% Saline	75	0	75	0	150	
1.26% Bicarbonate	150	0	0	0	300	Bicarbonate (HCO_3^-) 150 mmol/L
NORMAL VALUE	135–145	3.5–5.5	95–105		280–295	

ELECTROLYTE ABNORMALITIES

Electrolyte abnormalities can be life threatening and their management depends on the speed of onset of the electrolyte derangement and the patient's existing co-morbidities. Electrolytes are important in many of the reactions in the human body, such as muscle contraction and conduction of action potentials, thus their derangement can cause widespread, and not always obvious, clinical signs and symptoms. Electrolyte imbalance is usually diagnosed in the lab, but clinical signs (such as absent reflexes or peripheral oedema) and other investigations (such as tall T waves on the ECG) may point to an underlying defect which needs to be investigated and ruled out or treated.

As previously mentioned, electrolyte distribution varies greatly inside and outside the cells. The urea and electrolyte (U+E) test results only represent the **serum** plasma values of electrolytes and it is important to remember the distribution of electrolytes throughout the body (see Table 2.4 for electrolyte composition). Electrolyte composition is directly related to the water content and pH of the fluid. Electrolytes are in a fine balance with each other, and one electrolyte abnormality can result in an abnormality of another electrolyte. Electrolyte disturbances are rarely a single-electrolyte issue.

Table 2.4 Table of electrolyte composition per compartment

Electrolytes	Intracellular compartment	Interstitial compartment	Intravascular compartment
Sodium	10	144	140
Potassium	160	4	4
Magnesium	13	0.5	1
Calcium	2	114	102
Phosphate	57	1	1
Bicarbonate	8	30	26
Protein	55	0	16

Source: Adapted from National Institute for Health and Care Excellence, CG174 Intravenous Fluid Therapy in Adults in Hospital. Manchester, UK: NICE, 2013. Available from https://www.nice.org.uk/guidance/cg174 Reproduced with permission.

The path from recognising electrolyte abnormalities to successful treatment includes the following:

1. Recognition – ensure biochemistry results are accurate and for the correct patient.
2. Assess patient's fluid status and for any clinical signs of the electrolyte abnormality.
3. Treat any life-threatening signs and symptoms immediately. For example:
   a. Severe acute hypo/hypernatremia.
   b. Hyperkalaemia
   c. Hypokalaemia

4. Order appropriate investigations.

   a. U+E
   b. Calcium, phosphate and magnesium
   c. ECG – especially for potassium and magnesium abnormalities
   d. Urinary and serum paired osmolarities
   e. Urinary sodium and potassium

5. Try to diagnose the underlying cause and treat.

6. Manage the electrolyte abnormality with IV or oral replacement or diet.

7. Repeat U+E to ensure the electrolyte abnormality has been corrected at the appropriate rate and to the appropriate serum value (Table 2.4).

REMEMBER

- Biochemistry values are **serum values**. They do not represent the total body content of the given electrolyte.
- Rapid changes can occur as electrolytes shift into and out of cells. For example, hyperkalaemia is treated by encouraging potassium into the cells with insulin and salbutamol.

Sodium abnormalities

Sodium is primarily an ECF cation and it determines the body's water content. Sodium value from the U+E test results represents the relative SERUM value; it does not provide the total content of body sodium. Furthermore, sodium values are dependent on the body's water content, for example a hypovolaemic hypernatraemia patient and a hypervolaemia hyponatremia patient might actually have the same total sodium but these patients will present with very different clinical pictures. It is sodium's role, as the main active osmole (apart from albumin and other proteins) to determine body water content but in turn sodium content is affected by the solvent (water) it is dissolved in. Thus, assessment of a patient's sodium status is never complete without the fluid status (water).

Hyponatraemia

Mild 130 – 135 mmol/L
Intermediate 129 – 125 mmol/L
Severe <125 mmol/L

Sodium abnormalities are normally grouped according to a patient's fluid status, due to the effects of sodium on water content and vice versa. As mentioned, sodium is the main ECF and will affect water content inside and out of the cell. Sodium abnormalities can cause cell swelling and this is most important in the brain. Brain cells are contained within the skull and their swelling can result in damage and cell death due to the limited space for expansion.

The speed of onset of hyponatremia is crucial in assessment and management of hyponatremia. Acute hyponatremia is a sudden decrease in serum sodium levels (<48 hours). Chronic and insidious (>48 hours) hyponatremia results in slowly changing osmolality and can be asymptomatic. Alternatively, it can result in confusion and cognitive decline, as well as gait instability and falls. *NICE* guidelines on hyponatremia are very informative and thorough; we have based our approach on the 2015 guidelines.

Hypovolemic hyponatremia

Results from LOSS of SODIUM and WATER, causes are as follows:

- Gastrointestinal losses: Diarrhoea and vomiting
- Excessive diuretic use
- Hyperglycaemia due to osmotic diuresis
- Haemorrhage
- Adrenocortical insufficiency
- Polyuria during recovery after acute kidney injury
- Burns
- Third-space losses, such as pancreatitis and bowel obstruction

Euvolemic hyponatremia

Results from LOSS of SODIUM but normal water, causes are as follows:

- Inappropriate antidiuretic hormone secretion (SIADH)
- Psychogenic polydipsia

- Hyperglycaemia: When glucose becomes an active osmole
- Hypothyroidism
- Chronic alcohol excess

Hypervolemic hyponatremia

Results from EXCESS WATER but normal sodium, causes are as follows:

- Heart failure
- Liver failure
- Low albumin
- Renal failure with decreased urine output

Drug causes of hyponatremia

Medication will often, but not always, cause hyponatremia due to increased secretion of ADH. The most common drug causes are the following:

- Diuretics: Thiazides are the most common cause (20% of patients in the community on thiazide diuretics will have a mild hyponatremia).
- Nonsteroidal anti-inflammatory drug (NSAIDs): In combination with dehydration due to exacerbating the ADH renal effect.
- Carbamazepine due to increase in ADH secretion.
- Selective serotonin reuptake inhibitors (SSRIs).
- Some antipsychotics: Haloperidol and phenothiazine.

Approach to assessing hyponatremia:

1. Acute or chronic.
2. Severity: mild, moderate or severe: Is the patient symptomatic?
3. If mild is there an obvious cause of hyponatremia? → Treat appropriately.
4. Patient's fluid status: Hypovolaemia, euvolaemia or hypervolaemia.
5. Serum osmolality.
   a. If low (<275 Osm/kg) → true hyponatremia.
   b. If within normal range (275–295 Osm/kg) → investigate pseudo-hyponatremia as a cause due to excess proteins or lipid.
   c. If high (>295 Osm/kg) → another osmole apart from sodium is the cause of high osmolality, investigate hyperglycaemia as a cause.

6. Urine osmolality.

   a. Review urine osmolality in the context of urinary sodium and patient's volume status.

   b. See *NICE* guidelines on hyponatremia from March 2015 for the full overview of investigations and how to apply them to assessment.

Signs and symptoms
- Asymptomatic
- Headache
- Confusion
- Drowsiness
- Myoclonic jerks and seizures
- Coma

Management
- Correct sodium slowly: 0.5–1 mmol/L/hr to avoid osmotic demyelination syndrome; in severe cases, an even slower rate can be applied.
- Monitor serum sodium closely.
- Stop exacerbating medication.
- Management should be under direct senior guidance, as this can be a medical emergency and patients can develop osmotic demyelination syndrome. Severe hyponatremia needs close monitoring in an HDU setting. Some management strategies include the following:
  - **Mild and asymptomatic**: Monitor only
  - **In severe**: Hypertonic saline, under senior guidance
  - **Hypervolaemia/SIADH**: Water restriction, as low as 500 mL/day
  - **Hypovolaemia**: 0.9% saline until ECF is restored

Hypernatremia
Sodium >145 mmol/L

Sodium content is linked to water content in the body; hypernatremia always results in hyperosmolar states since sodium is the main ECF osmole, drawing water into the ECF. Although hypernatremia can exist in hypo/eu/hypervolaemia states, it generally indicates a decrease of water and, as a result, increased sodium in comparison. The human body tries to compensate for this via the thirst mechanism, and when this mechanism is impaired or can no longer compensate, exaggerated sodium values are seen.

Causes
- Cranial diabetes insipidus (DI) (ADH deficiency)
- Nephrogenic DI
- Water loss: Burns, heat stroke and hyperventilation
- Iatrogenic: Hypertonic IVF, large quantities of isotonic sodium containing IVF and sodium containing medication
- Inadequate water intake: Due to loss of consciousness, immobility and loss of thirst

Signs and symptoms
- Thirst
- Nausea and vomiting
- Confusion
- Convulsions
- Polyuria and polydipsia in diabetes mellitus

Treatment
- Normalise sodium gradually at 0.5–1 mmol/L/hr.
- Monitor sodium levels regularly to ensure slow increase.
- Oral intake: water replacement via oral route in hypovolaemia slowly (>0.5 mmol/L/hr).
- IVF: 5% glucose or 0.45% saline should be used with caution and under senior guidance only or in HDU setting.
- Diuretics can be used to treat iatrogenic causes in patients with normal renal function.
- Stop exacerbating and nephrotoxic medication.

Specific
- Cranial DI: Desmopressin can be used to replace ADH under senior or expert instruction only.
- DI in general will need large amounts of fluid.

Potassium abnormalities

Potassium is the main ICF cation and helps to determine the body's pH as it is exchanged for H^+ ions across the cell membrane and in the kidneys. As the primary positive ions inside the cells, potassium determines the cell membrane resting potential and its movement across the membrane is important in determining the action and resting membrane potential (RMP). Clinically, this is of particular importance in the cardiac cells and potassium abnormalities can result in life-threatening arrhythmias.

To understand the management of potassium abnormalities, it is necessary to know the causes of potassium shift in and out of the intravascular space. Potassium is naturally gained from the diet and its plasma levels rise due to the shift of potassium out of the cells. Potassium excretion is mainly controlled by three mechanisms: renal losses, gastrointestinal losses (such as vomiting and diarrhoea) and movement into the cells.

Thus, potassium abnormalities are caused by the following:

1. **Renal source**: Aldosterone causes excretion of potassium and H^+ ions in exchange for sodium in the collecting duct.

   a. Potassium loss: Increased aldosterone and alkalosis (due to excretion of H^+ ions).

   b. Potassium gain: Decreased aldosterone and acidosis.

2. **Gastrointestinal source**: Gastrointestinal juices are rich in potassium and their losses result in decreased potassium.

   a. Stomach: Can result in 10 mmol/L of potassium loss.

   b. Diarrhoea: Can result in 10–30 mmol/L of potassium loss.

   c. Small intestine: Ileus can result in potassium shift into the 'third space' and result in decreased serum potassium.

3. **Cellular shift**: Most of the body's potassium is inside the cells and vast changes in serum values can be seen when potassium goes in and out of the cells.

   a. Decreased serum potassium (shift into the cells): Insulin, salbutamol (β-adrenergic receptors stimulators) and theophylline.

   b. Increased serum potassium (shift out of the cells): Acidosis (potassium ions are exchanged for H^+ ions), α-adrenergic receptor stimulators, cell death resulting in release of potassium (e.g. gut ischaemia).

Hypokalaemia
Potassium <3.5 mmol/L

Hypokalaemia can develop suddenly, for example with diarrhoea and vomiting, and needs urgent treatment to ensure arrhythmias do not develop (cardiac patients are at particular risk). Alternatively, hypokalaemia can have a slow insidious onset, for example with diuretic use, or iatrogenic due to IVF replacement without potassium when using 0.9% saline or 5% dextrose.

Causes
- Dietary insufficiency: inadequate intake from food, e.g. patients that are NBM or intubated and ventilated
- Renal disease: renal tubular damage, renal tubular acidosis, rare renal syndromes (Bartter's, Gitelman's, Liddle's)
- Hyperaldosteronism secondary to: Conn's syndrome, Cushing's syndrome, heart failure, liver failure, nephrotic syndrome
- Losses from the gut: vomiting, diarrhoea, ileus, overproductive stomas
- Potassium shift into the cells: salbutamol, theophylline, insulin, alkalosis
- Iatrogenic: thiazides, loop diuretics, IVF without potassium supplementation (0.9% saline, 5% dextrose)

Signs and symptoms
- Asymptomatic
- Nausea and vomiting
- Ileus and constipation
- Atrial and ventricular atopic beats, and serious arrhythmias
- ECG: Flattened T waves
- Muscle weakness (<2.5 mmol/L)
- Paraesthesia
- Hyponatremia and associated signs and symptoms
- Increased risk of digoxin toxicity

Treatment
- Correct K slowly; fast administration of potassium can be very dangerous. Patients may also require continuous ECG monitoring depending on the rate of correction.

- Oral replacement if mild: Potassium supplements, e.g. Sando K (contains 470 mg [12 mmol] of potassium and 285 mg [8 mmol] of chloride per tablet).
- IVF potassium replacement: 20 or 40 mmol added to 1 L of 0.9% saline: Maximum 40 mmol in 1-L IVF over 4 hours.
- Ensure magnesium (Mg) is within range and replace if low (intractable hypokalaemia may be due to Mg deficiency).
- Severe hypokalaemia may require continuous cardiac monitoring.

Specific

- Hyperaldosteronism: Spironolactone or eplerenone under senior direction only.
- Natural deficiency: Increase dietary intake or oral supplements, e.g. Sando K.

Hyperkalaemia

Potassium >5.5 mmol/L

Potassium >6.5mmol/L in an emergency

Hyperkalaemia can be a medical emergency, as very quickly it can result in arrhythmias, cardiac arrest and death. Potassium is the major ICF cation and as such contributes the most to the RMP. With increased ECF potassium, the RMP becomes more positive and the cells become more easily excitable. This is of particular importance in the myocardial cells, because if they become more excitable it can result in arrhythmias. In patients who are post-MI or prone to arrhythmias it is desirable to keep potassium above 4.0 mmol/L.

Causes

- Renal: acute kidney injury, deteriorating chronic renal failure, acute or chronic renal failure
- Potassium shift out of cells: cell death (gut ischaemia), exercise (e.g. after marathons), DKA, acidosis
- Hormonal: aldosterone deficiency, Addison's disease
- Iatrogenic: angiotensin converting enzyme (ACE) inhibitors, spironolactone, NSAIDs, Heparin
- Blood transfusion

Signs and symptoms
- Asymptomatic
- Anxiety
- Diarrhoea and abdominal cramps
- ECG changes: Tall T waves, widened QRS complex
- Muscle weakness
- Paraesthesia
- Signs of metabolic acidosis: Kussmaul's breathing

Treatment
- Calcium gluconate 10%: 10 mL over several minutes if there are ECG changes, as it is cardio-protective but does not decrease overall body potassium
- Stop any medication causing hyperkalaemia
- Correct severe acidosis: 1.26% sodium bicarbonate

Decrease potassium

- Insulin–dextrose infusion: 10 units of insulin and 50% dextrose 50 mL over 30 minutes, check blood glucose
- Salbutamol nebulisers or salbutamol infusion (0.5 mg of salbutamol in 5% dextrose 100 mL)
- Haemodialysis if hyperkalaemia is not responding to medical management

Magnesium abnormalities

Magnesium is an ICF cation, primarily found in the cells of bones. However, magnesium balance is not related to bone reabsorption (as in phosphate) but mainly to dietary intake and renal excretion. Although not routinely measured, magnesium is very important for many of the essential reactions in the body. Magnesium is used for treatment of acute exacerbation of asthma and to protect against seizures in pre-eclampsia.

Hypomagnesaemia
Magnesium <0.7 mmol/L

Hypomagnesaemia can be common in malnourished patients and those with decreased oral intake, for example intubated patients in

ITU. Hypomagnesaemia can also cause or exacerbate other electrolyte disturbances, such as hypokalaemia and hypocalcaemia, so should be corrected alongside deficiencies in these electrolytes.

Causes
- Dietary insufficiency: Malnutrition and chronic alcohol excess
- Renal losses: DKA, SIADH, hyperaldosteronism
- Losses from the gut: Diarrhoea, fistulae
- Pancreatitis
- Iatrogenic: Aminoglycosides, digoxin, loop diuretics, thiazide diuretics, proton pump inhibitors

Signs and symptoms
- Weakness and fatigue
- Confusion
- Tremor
- Ataxia
- Hyper-reflexia
- Irritability, confusion, hallucinations
- Epileptic seizures
- ECG changes: Flattened and broad T waves, prolonged QT interval

Treatment
- Magnesium replacement: usually with a magnesium infusion
- Stop medication causing decreased magnesium, e.g. diuretics

Hypermagnesaemia
Magnesium >1.1 mmol/L

Hypermagnesaemia is mainly caused by excessive intake of magnesium in patients with renal failure that are not able to excrete the ion. For example, this can occur with aggressive magnesium replacement or medication containing magnesium (laxatives and enemas).

Causes
- Renal failure: AKI or chronic renal failure
- Addison's disease (acute adrenocortical failure)
- Iatrogenic: Magnesium-containing medication, e.g. antacids
- Iatrogenic: Magnesium replacement infusions for pre-eclampsia

Signs and symptoms

- Weakness
- Hypo-reflexia: Especially useful when assessing patients with pre-eclampsia on a magnesium infusion
- Cardiac arrhythmias
- Respiratory paralysis
- Narcosis

Treatment

- Stop precipitating medication
- As with hyperkalaemia:
  - 10% calcium gluconate 10 mL: Unlike in hyperkalaemia it is used to counter the magnesium effect on nerve cells
  - Insulin–dextrose to drive Mg into cells
- Diuretics in patients with good renal function
- Haemodialysis (with magnesium-free dialysate)

Phosphate abnormalities

Phosphate is primarily an ICF anion mostly found in bone cells. Serum phosphate is only a minute percentage of total body phosphate, but since serum phosphate is in continuous equilibrium with total phosphate it can be used as an indicator of phosphate levels. Phosphate balance is maintained by oral intake, release from bones and renal reabsorption and excretion. It is an important electrolyte for fundamental reactions and is found in nucleic acid. Phosphate levels are closely linked with calcium, sodium and vitamin D.

Hypophosphataemia
Phosphate <0.8 mmol/L

Phosphate is mainly an ICF and shift into the cells can cause low serum phosphate levels.

Causes

- Dietary insufficiency: malnutrition and vomiting
- Vitamin D deficiency
- Hyperparathyroidism and after parathyroidectomy
- Re-feeding syndrome
- Dent's disease

Signs and symptoms

- Lethargy
- Muscle weakness and pain
- Decreased coordination
- Decreased cardiac contraction
- Diaphragmatic weakness
- Confusion
- Memory loss
- Hallucinations
- Convulsions

Treatment

- Oral phosphate replacement in mild cases
- Calcitriol
- Intravenous phosphate in severe cases

Hyperphosphataemia
Phosphate >1.15 mmol/L

Phosphate is excreted in the kidneys and therefore chronic renal failure is a major cause of hyperphosphataemia. As phosphate is one of the primary intracellular ions, its release from the cells is another cause of hyperphosphotaemia. Excess phosphate can result in calcification of vessels and joints due to calcium phosphate.

Causes

- Chronic kidney failure
- Phosphate shift out of cells: rhabdomyolysis and tumour-lysis
- Iatrogenic: enemas containing phosphate

Signs and symptoms

- Asymptomatic
- Anorexia
- Nausea and vomiting
- Itching
- Hyper-reflexia
- Calcification of blood vessels and joints

Treatment

- If not severe, no treatment may be required
- Phosphate binders, e.g. magnesium antacids
- Dialysis

DEFINITIONS OF ESSENTIAL CONCEPTS

Some revision of basic biochemical concepts is crucial to understand the movement of fluids and electrolytes. We will look at the definitions of the essential forces responsible for water and electrolyte distribution throughout the body.

Osmosis: The movement of solutes across a semi-permeable membrane, from a solution with a lower concentration of particles (osmoles) to a solution with a higher concentration. In the human body, the solvent is water and the semi-permeable membranes are the cell membranes and capillary vessel walls. Water travels freely throughout all fluid compartments and is distributed via osmosis. Osmosis of water depends on the main osmole concentrations. Measurement of osmotic pressure is expressed in millimetres of mercury. This is a measure of the hydrostatic pressure needed to stop the osmosis of water.

Osmoles: Particles within a solution that cannot cross the semi-permeable membrane and hence exert an osmotic effect. The particles are measured in moles once dissolved in a solution, irrespective of whether they are atoms or molecules. Molecules that become ionised when dissolved (that is the compound dissociates into its components that have an electric charge once in solution) will have an effective osmolality depending on the number of particles they dissociate into.

Osmoles in the body: these include sodium, glucose, mannitol and sorbitol. Sodium is the main solute as it is the major ECF cation and cannot freely enter the cells. Glucose becomes relevant in diabetes mellitus because, unlike in health, it is not absorbed by cells and thus will have an osmotic effect on water.

Osmolality: The result of solute concentration. The number of particles within the solution will determine its osmolality, irrespective of their size. It is the measure of osmoles per kilogram of solvent (Osm/kg). It is not affected by temperature so it is often the preferred value when dealing with serum values.

Osmolarity: Measure of the osmoles of solute per litre of a solution (Osm/L). Is often used in IVF composition. However, the two definitions are very similar for plasma.

Plasma osmolarity = 2 × (Sodium + Potassium) + Glucose + Urea

Osmolar gap: OSM (measured) – OSM (calculated). If this is bigger than 10 it suggests the presence of another solute not measured, typically due to an excess of alcohol, sugars, proteins or lipids in the blood.

Tonicity: This is the force which moves water between compartments, across the semi-permeable membrane, and it is caused by the combined effect of all solutes within a single compartment. Tonicity is the 'effective osmolality'. It is the concentration of particles in a solution and the effect this has on the diffusion of water. In the human body, the tonicity and osmolality effects are the same. Essentially, it is about movement of water across a semi-permeable membrane. So, increased tonicity means an increased concentration of osmoles in a solution and this attracts water from the neighbouring compartment. Tonicity stimulates thirst and ADH release.

- *Hypertonicity* reduces the cell volume and *hypotonicity* expands the cell volume due to the osmosis of water (more water = bigger size).
- *Hypertonicity* means that water will diffuse INTO the compartment and thus a reduction of water in the neighbouring compartment.
- *Hypotonicity* means water will diffuse OUT of the compartment and thus cause an increase in water in the neighbouring compartment. These terms are especially used in reference to IVFs.

CONCLUSION

In this chapter, we have reviewed the wide range of topics that underpin the physiological basis of water and electrolytes in the human body, and the IVFs and electrolytes we use to replace them when needed.

First, we have covered the water composition of the human body in the different compartments which should always be at the forefront of your mind when assessing a patient's fluid status. The basics of movement of water throughout the body were outlined to help you understand the impact of prescribing different IVFs and electrolytes. To help with your fluid assessment, average human water inputs and outputs are highlighted and you can refer back to Table 2.1 when needed. To further aid with your IVF prescribing daily human water and electrolyte requirements as per *NICE* guidelines are summarised in Table 2.2.

Second, we have summarised renal physiology. This is not a replacement for a dedicated physiology textbook, but we have outlined the main functions of the nephron. Furthermore, we have covered the kidneys' hormonal function with respect to water and electrolyte handling. Renal electrolyte handling was outlined for each electrolyte in order to provide you with some background knowledge when thinking about electrolytes.

Third, we have analysed IVF in both the subtypes (colloid and crystalloid) and individually. An in-depth overview of each IVF should be useful when debating which IVF to prescribe and hopefully should prompt you to tailor your prescribing, even on long night shifts. Specific uses of some IVFs and the need for prescribing by a senior were also highlighted.

Fourth, electrolyte abnormalities were summarised. Specific signs, symptoms, investigation and management of each electrolyte excess and deficit were covered.

Finally, we have expanded on some commonly used definitions. The grasp of these terms and their clinical application will not only aid you in better understanding this book but also more advanced texts and research on IVF should your interest take you further!

References

Government Safety Alert Regarding HES. Hydroxyethyl Starch (HES) Products – Increased Risk of Renal Dysfunction and Mortality. 2013. https://www.gov.uk/drug-device-alerts/drug-alert-hydroxyethyl-starch-hes-products-increased-risk-of-renal-dysfunction-and-mortality.

NICE Guideline. *Intravenous Fluid Therapy in Adults in Hospital.* 2013. https://www.nice.org.uk/guidance/cg174.

NICE Hyponatraemia Clinical Knowladge Summary. https://cks.nice.org.uk/hyponatraemia#!topicsummary.

Further reading

Anaesthesia UK. Summary of IV Fluids Composition. http://www.frca.co.uk/article.aspx?articleid=295.

British National Formulary (BNF). https://www.evidence.nhs.uk/formulary/bnf/current/9-nutrition-and-blood/92-fluids-and-electrolytes.

Eccles F. *Electrolytes Body Fluids and Acid Base Balance*. Kent, UK: Hodder and Stoughton, 1993.

E-Learning for Health: Anaesthesia: Physics and Statistics. http://www.e-lfh.org.uk/programmes/anaesthesia/

Fox S. *Human Physiology*, 12th Edition. New York, NY: McGraw-Hill, 2011.

Green JH. *Basic Clinical Physiology*, 3rd Edition. Oxford, UK: Oxford University Press, 1978.

Heitz UE and Horne MM. *Mosby's Pocket Guide Series: Fluid, Electrolyte and Acid-Base Balance*. St Louis, MO: Mosby, 2001.

Leach R. *Critical Care Medicine at a Glance*. Chichester, UK: John Wiley and Sons, 2009.

Oxford Medical Education. How to Prescribe IV Fluids. http://www.oxfordmedicaleducation.com /prescribing/iv-fluids/.

Preston RA. *Acid-Base, Fluids and Electrolytes Made Ridiculously Simple*. Miami, FL: MedMaster, 2002.

Smith KM. *Fluids and Electrolytes: A Conceptual Approach*, 2nd edition. Edinburgh, UK: Churchill Livingstone, 1991.

Spoors C and Kiff K. *Training in Anaesthesia the Essential Curriculum*. Oxford, UK: Oxford University Press, 2010.

Sweeney RM, McKendry RA and Bedi A. Perioperative Intravenous Fluid Therapy for Adults. *Ulster Medical Journal*, September 2013; 82(3): 171–178. http://www.ncbi.nlm.nih.gov/pmc/articles/PMC3913409 /pdf/umj0082-0171.pdf.

Willis L. *Just the Facts: Fluids and Electrolytes Made Incredibly Easy*. Philadelphia, PA: Lippincott Williams and Wilkins, 2005.

Yentis SM, Hirsch NP and Ip JK. *Anaesthesia and Intensive Care A-Z*, 5th Edition. London, UK: Elsevier Churchill Livingstone, 2013.

CHAPTER 3

Cardiac arrest and shock

INTRODUCTION

Emergency situations such as peri-arrest, cardiac arrest and shock require prompt recognition and action to prevent significant morbidity or indeed mortality. As a junior doctor, you may well be the first person on the scene in an inpatient setting and are expected to help resuscitate and stabilise the patient, as part of a multidisciplinary team. This is the time to put your emergency care training into practice; do not hesitate to participate, your contribution is invaluable.

Specifically, this chapter focuses on those emergency situations that require consideration of the most appropriate intravenous fluid (IVF) therapy to administer: cardiac arrest, hypovolaemic shock, sepsis and anaphylaxis. Comprehensive management of these conditions is beyond the scope of this book; instead we aim to improve your knowledge of the IVF therapy aspects of management.

ASSESSMENT

The assessment of the unwell or collapsed patient is the same in hospital and in community settings and allows you to quickly determine if urgent resuscitation including fluid resuscitation is required. This involves the 'ABCDE' approach, using the team to simultaneously check and address problems at each stage. Assess your surroundings, ensure it is safe to approach the patient, and shake and shout to determine whether they are able to respond or not.

Airway

Airway obstruction is the partial or complete limitation of the entry of air into the lungs. A state of altered consciousness (sepsis, drug toxicity), airway inflammation (asthma attack, anaphylaxis) or physical obstruction by inhaled objects could cause this medical emergency. There is a risk of hypoxaemia, irreversible damage to vital organs and death. Symptoms and signs of airway obstruction are listed in Table 3.1. Remove any large debris within easy reach, gently tilt the head backwards and lift the chin forwards to open the airway. If a neck injury is suspected, stabilise the neck but thrust the jaw forwards to maintain the airway. High-flow oxygen at 15 L/min should be commenced via a bag-valve mask and airway adjuncts can be used to maintain the airway in unconscious patients.

Table 3.1 Signs and symptoms of airway obstruction

Symptoms	Signs
• Abnormal or absent breath sounds • Choking sounds • Stridor • Wheeze	• See-saw pattern of respiration • Accessory muscle use • Central cyanosis • Oxygen saturation <92%

Breathing

Abnormal breathing can occur for several reasons including pulmonary oedema, severe pneumonia and tension pneumothorax. Determine if respiratory distress is present (Table 3.2), and look, listen and feel (<10 seconds) for signs of breathing. Inspect, percuss and auscultate the chest for clues to the underlying cause of respiratory distress.

Although the treatment of acute breathing problems depends on the underlying cause, all patients require high-flow oxygen to reduce the risk of hypoxaemia, respiratory arrest and death. Administer oxygen at 15 L/min via a bag-valve or pocket mask to maintain oxygen saturation greater than 92% and respiratory rate (RR) at 12–20 breaths/min. In those with known carbon dioxide retention secondary to chronic obstructive pulmonary disease (COPD), high oxygen levels may rarely lead to type II respiratory failure, so aim for oxygen saturation of 88%–92% instead. A 24% or 28% Venturi mask with a fixed flow rate can help with achieving these parameters. Review management and titrate oxygen flow rates in line with the patient's response to therapy, both clinically and on arterial blood gases (ABGs). Consider non-invasive ventilation if the patient tolerates it and does not require intubation.

Table 3.2   Signs and symptoms of respiratory distress

Symptoms	Signs
• Abnormal or absent breath sounds • Sweating • Rattling airway noises • Altered consciousness	• See-saw pattern of respiration • Accessory muscle use • Central cyanosis • Oxygen saturation <92% • Respiratory rate outside the normal range of 12–20 breaths/min • Bronchial breathing • Chest hyper-resonance or dullness • Tracheal deviation

Circulation

Assessing a patient's circulation refers to identifying haemodynamic collapse, otherwise known as circulatory failure; blood is either not being pumped around the body effectively or the amount of blood that is supplied to tissues is inadequate, leading to clinical manifestations of hypotension (see Table 3.3). Hypovolaemia (especially in haemorrhage) is a common cause of haemodynamic collapse and therefore should be considered and addressed quickly when faced with an acutely unwell patient. Whilst looking for the source of haemorrhage (overt or concealed), in the presence of hypotension, be sure to administer fluid challenge(s) (warm colloid, 500 mL stat or 250 mL if existing heart failure or trauma) to help replace lost intravascular fluid volume. If there is ongoing bleeding, crossmatch at least two units of red blood cells and consider instigating your hospital's major haemorrhage protocol; large volumes of lost blood need to be replaced with similar volumes of transfused blood components.

Arrhythmia, underlying structural cardiac disease, chronic heart failure and of course problems with breathing (e.g. tension pneumothorax) can also cause haemodynamic collapse. The pathophysiology of haemodynamic collapse is covered in more detail in the 'Hypovolaemic Shock' section of this chapter.

Treating circulatory failure is multi-factorial and depends on the underlying cause; however, universal resuscitation aims to replace lost intravascular fluid, control haemorrhage and restore systemic circulation. Attach a defibrillator or cardiac monitor to the patient as soon as possible after identifying circulatory failure and follow the advanced life support (ALS) algorithm (see Figure 3.1 later in the chapter), prioritising chest compressions (30 chest compressions: 2 rescue breaths for adults).

After the initial fluid challenge, reassess the patient, and check the blood pressure (BP), heart rate (HR), RR and temperature every 5–15 minutes. Aim to restore the patient's normal BP or a sustained level above 100/60 mmHg. Auscultate the chest for pulmonary crepitations suggestive of fluid overload. Adjust the rate of fluid infusion accordingly if this occurs. If acute coronary syndrome is suspected or confirmed, administer Aspirin 300 mg, Clopidogrel 300 mg, Oxygen 15 L/min, Nitroglycerine and IV Morphine (MONAC). Arrange percutaneous coronary intervention if there is ST-elevation or a new left bundle branch block present.

Table 3.3 Signs and symptoms of circulatory failure

Symptoms	Signs
• Pale, blue or mottled skin	• Capillary refill time (CRT) >2 seconds
• Grey mucosal surfaces in dark-skinned people	• Collapsed veins
• Altered consciousness	• Poorly palpable or bounding pulses
• Dizziness, pre-syncope	• Tachycardia or bradycardia
• Dyspnoea	• Arrhythmia
• Bleeding from mucosal or wound surfaces	• Heart murmur or diminished heart sounds
• Bleeding into wound drains, packs, incontinence pads	• Narrowed pulse pressure (<35–45 mmHg)
	• Low diastolic blood pressure (BP) (<50 mmHg)
	• Decreased urine output (<0.5 mL/kg/hr)

Disability

This involves determining the level of unconsciousness in an unwell patient and identifying and managing the underlying causes of this. Ensure that the 'ABC' aspects of assessment have been identified and properly treated before moving on to 'D'. Causes of altered consciousness include cerebral hypoperfusion, profound hypoxia, hypercapnia, hypoglycaemia, sedatives and opioid analgesia. A rapid initial assessment can be made using the 'AVPU' method or Glasgow Coma Scale (GCS). If the patient is unresponsive to all stimuli or scores eight or less on GCS, a severe injury is indicated, their airway needs to be protected (intubation) and further investigation is required.

Venous or arterial blood gas measurement of blood glucose is more reliable than capillary measurement in a collapsed or unwell patient. If less than 4 mmol/L, administer 50-mL doses of 10% glucose intravenously until the patient becomes conscious or 250 mL is given, whilst monitoring the blood glucose level.

Exposure

Whilst maintaining the patient's dignity, remove all outer clothing that impedes full patient assessment, remove wound dressings, inspect external surgical packs and roll the patient onto their sides. Aim to find more clues as to why the patient has deteriorated or become unconscious.

Once the initial 'ABCDE' assessment has been made and the patient is stable, further investigations such as an ABG, blood tests and imaging

> **REMEMBER**
>
> **4Hs and 4Ts**
>
> **Hypoxia:** Ventilate the patient with high-flow oxygen or via an advanced airway.
>
> **Hypovolaemia:** Often caused by haemorrhage. Replace intravascular fluid volume with fluids or blood components. Stop ongoing loss.
>
> **Hypo-/Hyperkalaemia** or other metabolic disturbances – quickly detect with an ABG/VBG. Reverse the disturbance and monitor cardiac activity in severe cases. IV calcium chloride in marked hyperkalaemia and hypocalcaemia.
>
> **Hypothermia:** Use a low-reading thermometer to detect and correct with a warming unit and warm IVF.
>
> Ensure you also pay attention to the patient's blood glucose level – many physicians advocate 'hypoglycaemia' as the fifth 'H'! It is easily missed but very easily treated.
>
> **Thrombosis:** May cause pulseless electrical activity, consider thrombolysis.
>
> **Tension pneumothorax:** Can occur after chest trauma or central line placement. Signs (absent breath sounds, deviated trachea, hyper-resonance) may indicate urgent thoracocentesis.
>
> **Tamponade (cardiac):** Confirmed by echocardiography, treated in severe cases by pericardiocentesis.
>
> **Toxins:** Have a low threshold for toxicology screens of blood, urine and hair. Consider antidotes and counter-agents such as naloxone and activated charcoal.
>
> Early consideration and treatment of one or more of these conditions can improve the chances of successful resuscitation.

can be conducted to help determine the cause of the patient's abnormal state. These can provide clues to reversible causes such as electrolyte disturbances, sepsis and hypoxia, otherwise known as the 4Hs and 4Ts. See Chapter 2 for more on electrolyte disturbances.

IVF for resuscitation

There is still wide variation in clinical practice when it comes to selecting the most appropriate type of IVF to administer in initial resuscitation. This may be due to a reliance on clinical experience and difficulty applying findings from clinical trials to everyday practice. In general, several review and consensus bodies are currently advocating the use of balanced crystalloids (e.g. Hartmann's, Plasmalyte) in resuscitation of acutely unwell patients. This advice is based on several large studies comparing outcomes when different types of fluids are used for initial resuscitation (SAFE, CHEST, CRYSTMAS, GIFTASUP, FEAST, included in the 'further reading' list at the end of this chapter). Balanced crystalloids have a similar ion composition to plasma, as they are isotonic (see Chapter 2 for definitions of these terms). This means that ions distribute within the intravascular space and through the semi-permeable capillary membrane into the interstitial space. There is no forward movement into cells as they do not penetrate the cell's lipid bilayer membrane. Balanced crystalloids distribute between the intravascular space and the interstitial space at a ratio of approximately 25%–75%, respectively.

Intravascular volume is restored by increasing the oncotic pressure in the intravascular space, i.e. water moves into the intravascular space, increasing circulatory volume. However, this effect is short-lived with balanced crystalloids, as the majority of fluid administered migrates into the interstitial space. This means that a larger volume of balanced crystalloid is required to initially replace the deficit in the intravascular volume and then to maintain it over time.

Balanced crystalloids are not always the ideal IVF to administer as initial resuscitation, so we will also discuss the pathophysiology behind common emergency situations that may indicate alternative IVF.

REMEMBER

IVF for initial resuscitation in an acutely unwell patient.
Secure a large bore cannula (14G or 16G).

Administer warm balanced crystalloids that contain sodium in the range 130–154 mmol/L (e.g. Hartmann's or Plasmalyte), with a bolus of 500 mL over 15 minutes or less (250-mL bolus if known to have chronic heart failure or elderly).

Review the implemented treatment within 15 minutes. Have the vital signs moved closer to normal levels? Or is there no improvement? Consider further fluid boluses, remaining watchful for signs of leakage into the interstitial space and fluid overload.

If the patient is persistently hypotensive, consider better intravascular fluid volume expansion with a colloid infusion (500 or 250 mL of e.g. Gelofusin) or replace blood lost with appropriate blood transfusions. Investigate and manage reversible causes of acute clinical deterioration.

Colloid or crystalloid?

So far, we have established that current expert advice is to administer a balanced crystalloid in bolus form as part of initial resuscitation of an acutely unwell patient. The aims of administering IVF (balanced crystalloid, colloid, both or blood components) in this situation are to restore intravascular fluid volume, stabilise haemodynamics and maintain tissue perfusion.

Reduction or loss of circulating fluid volume decreases venous return, preload and in turn cardiac output. This leads to clinical manifestations of hypotension and poor peripheral and eventually central perfusion. The initial IVF in this situation acts as a rapid plasma volume expander; oncotic pressure in the intravascular space increases, water is drawn in and circulating volume increases. Improved central venous pressure (CVP), cardiac output, stroke volume, BP and tissue perfusion follow.

On the whole, colloids are good plasma volume expanders; they contain large molecules that do not easily cross the semi-permeable capillary membrane and the volume required to replace the deficit of fluid is 1:1. The ratio of required volume of balanced crystalloid to volume of fluid lost is 3:1 in comparison. Infused colloids also stay within the intravascular space for a longer period of time than crystalloids do. When used for resuscitation, colloids can cause anaphylactic reactions or peripheral/pulmonary/cerebral oedema or heart failure, especially when used in excessive volumes. Oedema occurs later than in crystalloid use, but is more sustained. In sepsis, anaphylaxis, severe trauma and other forms of inflammation, the capillary vessel walls become leakier, allowing the colloid molecules to cross into the interstitial layer – oedema. Some studies have also shown an increased risk of mortality with the use of colloids in these situations – avoid using them. In addition, large volumes of some colloids (starches, dextran) can contribute to coagulopathy by interfering with platelet function, and clotting factor complexes, especially if clotting factors are depleted and not replaced – avoid using them.

Although more robust clinical trials have been conducted and meta-analysed recently, a common outcome measured is mortality; starch-based colloids used as resuscitation fluids have been associated with a higher risk of mortality and therefore their use is advised against. Starch-based colloids and gelatins are also advised against in severe sepsis and those at risk of acute kidney injury.

In summary, balanced crystalloids (Hartmann's, Plasmalyte) are now the recommended fluid of choice for initial resuscitation of an acutely unwell patient, where there is no ongoing bleeding. Gelatin-based colloids (Volplex, Gelofusin) are useful when there is ongoing bleeding, whilst waiting for replacement blood to arrive. Treat the patient individually; they may need more than one type of fluid to restore adequate circulation and tissue perfusion, and in varying amounts. Monitor electrolyte levels to avoid life-threatening imbalances. As always, review your implemented treatment quickly, consider additional measures and seek senior and multidisciplinary help.

CARDIAC ARREST

If a patient is found to be unresponsive, not breathing and without a pulse, they are in cardiac arrest; there is a sudden cessation of organised electrical activity and the heart stops pumping effectively enough to maintain circulation and tissue perfusion. This emergency situation requires prompt action to have any chance of restoring life (see Figure 3.1).

Cardiac arrest is more common in those with coronary heart disease or with other underlying structural or electrical cardiac problems. An exacerbation such as sepsis, electrolyte disturbances, ischaemia or pro-arrhythmic drugs may trigger cardiac arrest in those with existing cardiac conditions such as myocarditis, long QT syndrome and chronic heart failure. Alternatively, cardiac arrest can be non-cardiac

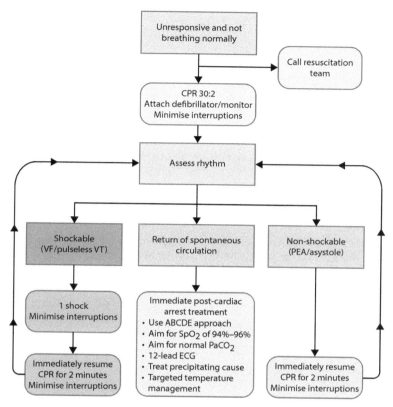

Figure 3.1 UK adult ALS algorithm. (From Resuscitation Council UK, *Adult Advanced Life Support,* 2016. https://www.resus.org.uk/resuscitation-guidelines/adult-advanced-life-support/. With Permission.)

in origin: near-drowning, pulmonary embolism or, drug toxicity for instance.

Essentially, the coronary and myocardial blood supply becomes disrupted by processes such as acute ischaemia in plaque rupture, electrolyte abnormalities or progressive worsening of cardiovascular function. These processes lead to un-coordinated electrical activity: ventricular fibrillation (VF), ventricular tachycardia (VT), asystole or pulseless electrical activity (PEA). In some cases, one abnormal heart rhythm can lead to another, such as sustained VT to VF.

Most hospitals have a rapid response team or similar; a multidisciplinary team tasked with assessing and stabilising the deteriorating patient and one in whom cardiac arrest has been identified. If resuscitation is successful, the most immediate threat is haemodynamic collapse. The circulatory system attempts to restore perfusion to vital organs, but in this fragile state, hypotension and circulatory failure can develop. Aim to maintain a balance between restoring intravascular volume, perfusing vital organs and avoiding excess strain on the heart. Balanced crystalloids are preferred in the initial stage, but the risk of ensuing cerebral or pulmonary oedema with large volumes may indicate an early switch to a colloid infusion instead. Aim for a mean arterial pressure (MAP) of 80–100 mmHg, CVP of 8–12 mmHg and urine output of ≥0.5 mL/kg/hr.

The inflammatory response to cardiac arrest often leads to peripheral vasodilatation severe enough to require treatment with vasopressors and inotropes. Vasopressors like noradrenaline work predominantly by increasing peripheral vasoconstriction and thus peripheral vascular resistance to maintain cardiac output and circulation. An inotrope like dobutamine acts on β1 receptors to increase the force of cardiac contractility and therefore cardiac output and circulation. Other factors to consider post–cardiac arrest are oxygenation, ventilation, correction of electrolyte disturbances and therapeutic cooling (to help minimise hypoxic-ischaemic brain injury). Note that decisions to use inotropes or vasopressors or therapeutic cooling are universally expected to be made by senior clinicians with the involvement of the high dependency/intensive care team. The patient is going to require close monitoring and is therefore often nursed in a high dependency, critical or intensive care setting anyway.

REMEMBER

IVF for initial resuscitation in a patient surviving cardiac arrest

Balanced crystalloids are preferred in the initial stage, but monitor the patient's response closely and alter the volume and type of administered fluid as necessary.

Aim for a mean arterial pressure (MAP) of 80–100 mmHg and urine output of ≥0.5 mL/kg/hr. Some clinicians still aim for central venous pressure (CVP) of 8–12 mmHg.

SEVERE SEPSIS AND SEPTIC SHOCK

Sepsis features systemic inflammation secondary to infection, the severity of which varies and can be fatal. Septic shock is a form of distributive shock whereby peripheral vasodilatation is impaired by the inflammatory process. The following criteria help to identify these conditions:

- **Severe inflammatory response syndrome (SIRS) criteria:**
  - Temperature >38°C or <36°C
  - Pulse >90 bpm
  - RR >20 breaths/min or $PaCO_2$ <32 mmHg
  - White cell count >12,000/mm³ or <4,000/mm³
- **Sepsis criteria (SIRS + source of infection):** Suspected or identified source of infection
- **Severe sepsis criteria (organ dysfunction, hypotension or hypoperfusion):** Lactic acidosis, systolic BP <90 mmHg or drop ≥40 mmHg from normal
- **Septic shock criteria:** Severe sepsis with hypotension despite adequate fluid resuscitation
- **Multiple organ dysfunction syndrome criteria:** Evidence of ≥2 organs failing

The *Surviving Sepsis* guidance is now commonly used in most developed countries and aims to help clinicians identify and manage sepsis effectively, to reduce the incidence of significant morbidity and mortality from this treatable condition.

Infection or inflammation causes injury or death of cells, which coupled with the release of both pro- and anti-inflammatory mediators could lead to organ dysfunction and death; the body's defence mechanisms become overwhelmed. Circulatory dysfunction is common in sepsis and occurs via the following mechanisms:

- **Vasodilation:** Vasoactive mediators such as nitric oxide and cytokines relax vascular smooth muscle, capillaries become leakier and endothelial cells are damaged.
- **Hypotension**: Systemic vascular resistance is reduced, although not uniformly across vascular beds. Hypotension in sepsis does not respond to sympathomimetic vasopressors in the same way as

occurs in other causes of hypotension, perhaps due to endothelial damage. Vasopressin, however, does work.

- **Intravascular fluid redistribution:** The permeability of the capillary endothelium increases, allowing abnormal transport of ions and water across gradients. Intravascular fluid volume reduces (hypovolaemia) whilst interstitial fluid volume increases.

- **Ventricular function:** The myocardium becomes depressed, systole is not as forceful and the myocardium is more lax in diastole. Initially, tachycardia becomes a compensatory mechanism to help maintain cardiac output (Starling's mechanism), but over time, this diminishes.

- **Tissue hypo-perfusion:** Injury to cells and the increased permeability of capillary walls impairs the delivery of oxygen to tissues and therefore their normal function is affected; no organ is spared the possibility of this phenomenon, which can be irreversible.

Use the 'ABCDE' approach to help recognise sepsis, then start initial resuscitation quickly, aiming to stabilise the patient within the first 6 hours. Early goal-directed therapy involves following particular protocols that enable MAP ≥65 mmHg, urine output ≥0.5 mL/kg/hr and if available, central venous oxygen saturation of 70%. Lactate levels can also be used as a measure of response to resuscitation, as this normalises as resuscitation succeeds. Antibiotics should be administered; follow your local protocol when making a choice. The source of infection should be identified and attempts should be made to limit the spread of infection; change lines and catheters, and isolate if necessary.

Balanced crystalloids are the IVF of choice in resuscitation of sepsis: boluses of 500 mL or 250 mL in chronic heart failure or the elderly, or 30 mL/kg within 15 minutes. Stay with the patient, if the bolus works, an improvement in hypotension, tachycardia and RR should occur. Further fluid challenges, vasopressors and inotropes may be required to achieve the patient's measured goals. Seek the input of your seniors and the high dependency/intensive care team.

REMEMBER

IVF for initial resuscitation in a patient identified as having sepsis

Administer warm balanced crystalloids as a bolus of 500 mL over 15 minutes or less. 250-mL bolus if known to have chronic heart failure or elderly. 30 mL/kg is recommended by the *Surviving Sepsis* guidelines.

Consider vasopressors and inotropes early in severe sepsis and septic shock.

Aim for a MAP ≥65 mmHg, urine output ≥0.5 mL/kg/hr, reducing lactate levels, and if available, central venous oxygen saturation of 70%.

ANAPHYLACTIC SHOCK

Anaphylaxis is an acute, severe, life-threatening, generalised or systemic hypersensitivity reaction mediated by the immune system. The majority of reactions involve IgE-dependent mechanisms, such as those triggered by foods, medications, insect stings and latex. Other reactions may be independent of IgE (IgG-dependent, clotting cascade activation), idiopathic or non-immunological; exercise, temperature extremes, contrast agents inducing a sudden massive mast cell or basophil degranulation without immunoglobulin presence.

Overall, anaphylaxis is a form of both distributive and hypovolaemic shock whereby multiple organs become compromised, especially the heart, circulatory system and lungs; circulatory collapse or respiratory arrest can occur if not treated promptly. Capillary permeability is increased by inflammatory processes, resulting in massive fluid shifts into the interstitial space, intravascular volume depletion and hypotension. There is reduced venous return and depressed myocardial contractility, which may progress to myocardial ischaemia and arrhythmias. The body tries to compensate for massive fluid shifts by releasing catecholamines and other vasoconstrictors to increase peripheral vascular resistance; however, shock can still persist if intravascular fluid volume is not restored. Tissue perfusion is decreased, which may lead to more widespread end-organ damage.

Symptoms may be non-specific, but the patient becomes rapidly unwell, requiring assessment with the 'ABCDE' approach and then appropriate resuscitation. Symptoms may include airway obstruction, facial swelling, itching, wheeze, hives/wheals and confusion. The onset of symptoms is often within minutes to hours of exposure to a trigger, although in some cases, this can take several weeks. Most commonly, symptoms appear, intensify, peak and then wane; however, in some cases, there may be a biphasic or prolonged reaction. Patients can deteriorate very quickly making anaphylaxis a challenging situation to manage.

Immediate treatment involves removing the antigen (e.g. stopping the antibiotic infusion), calling for help, 'ABCDE' assessment, intramuscular (IM) or IV adrenaline, high-flow oxygen and volume resuscitation with crystalloids. Give a fluid challenge of 500–1000-mL Hartmann's/Plasmalyte stat: larger volumes may be required, especially if there is slow improvement despite adrenaline. This implies ongoing intravascular volume depletion despite peripheral vasoconstriction.

In selecting a balanced crystalloid over other fluids, consider the following points:

- No benefit has been shown of colloids like gelatins over crystalloids such as Hartmann's and 0.9% normal saline in anaphylaxis resuscitation. There is a potential risk of anaphylaxis to infused colloid, especially in the immune system's already hyper-alert state.

- Dextrose rapidly migrates from the intravascular space to the interstitial space, therefore not correcting hypotension.

Antihistamines (offer relief from itching and urticaria), steroids (reduce the late-phase response and risk of prolonged anaphylaxis) and oxygen-nebulised bronchodilators (offer relief from bronchospasm) are also administered.

REMEMBER

IVF for initial resuscitation in a patient identified as having anaphylaxis

Identify and address the trigger for anaphylaxis, call for help and administer adrenaline as soon as possible.

Large volumes (several litres) of balanced crystalloid (Hartmann's or Plasmalyte) may be required to maintain intravascular fluid volume. Start with a bolus of 500–1000 mL stat, review the observations within 15 minutes and administer more as necessary.

Colloids may trigger anaphylaxis and have not been shown to have any significant benefit over crystalloids in resuscitation from anaphylaxis.

HYPOVOLAEMIC SHOCK

Hypovolaemic shock arises as a result of loss of blood or salt and water from plasma. This can therefore be haemorrhagic or non-haemorrhagic in origin. Haemorrhagic causes include trauma, gastrointestinal (GI) bleeding, ruptured aneurysm and post-partum haemorrhage. Non-haemorrhagic causes include loss through the GI tract (diarrhoea, stoma output), renal system (diabetes insipidus, osmotic diuresis), skin (burns) or into the third space in the post-operative state. This text will focus on haemorrhagic shock.

There is a phased response to hypovolaemia, depending on the volume of fluid or blood lost and the time scale. Initially, the body tries to compensate; baroreceptors detect the reduced intravascular volume and trigger the release of catecholamines (peripheral vasoconstriction). This increases intravascular fluid volume (leading to increased preload), systemic vascular resistance (measured as afterload), BP and therefore tissue perfusion. Cardiac sympathetic drive also increases to produce tachycardia and increased cardiac output. Other early compensatory mechanisms include movement of fluid from the intracellular and interstitial spaces to the intravascular space.

As further intravascular fluid volume depletion occurs with advancing hypovolaemic shock, the compensatory mechanisms become overwhelmed; systemic vascular resistance and BP are not well maintained, and profound hypotension occurs. Vasopressors may be used to address this if there is no improvement despite restoring intravascular fluid volume. The initial tachycardia becomes bradycardia, and the force of ventricular contractility diminishes. Haemorrhagic shock in particular causes a significant lactic acidosis; reduced tissue perfusion means oxygen is in short supply, anaerobic metabolism occurs, and insufficient ATP is produced leading to cell death and end-organ dysfunction.

Compensation for hypovolaemia shifts to a longer term phase with a reduction in glomerular filtration rate, salt and water reabsorption (mediated by aldosterone, vasopressin) and increased erythropoiesis (more red blood cells providing increased oxygen-carrying capacity). These effects are thought to occur once effective arterial blood volume reduces by approximately 30%. The patient's clinical status changes, and signs and symptoms of hypovolaemia and end-organ dysfunction develop; the situation can deteriorate into circulatory collapse and cardiac arrest if not treated promptly.

The aims of resuscitation in haemorrhagic shock are to stop the bleeding and restore intravascular fluid volume, tissue perfusion and oxygen delivery to prevent irreversible organ damage and death.

In haemorrhagic shock, fluid challenges of warm, balanced crystalloids can still be used initially, but then follow this with red blood cells as soon as possible or with a colloid if there is a delay. Remember that 0.9% normal saline can cause hyperchloraemic acidosis and renal impairment, so avoid its use in large amounts. Consider transfusion of blood components (see Chapter 6) early in the process of resuscitation, especially if haemorrhage has not been stemmed yet. Remember that the volume of replacement blood should match the volume of lost blood; if 2 L of blood has been lost, this is the volume that should be replaced. In the immediate period after haemorrhage, there will not be a drop in haemoglobin count; emptying half of a bucket of blood will leave you with the same concentration of blood in your bucket, just at a lower volume. A drop in haemoglobin count occurs over time, when dilution takes place by physiological fluid shifts between compartments or when intravascular fluid is administered.

Do not wait for laboratory results of full blood count (FBC) and clotting profiles before requesting cryoprecipitate, fresh frozen plasma or platelet transfusions. If there is ongoing bleeding, clotting factor replacement is essential, before disseminated intravascular coagulation (DIC) develops. Thromboelastography-guided transfusion is a newer concept that uses real-time collation of coagulation test results to determine the performance of the clotting system and therefore guide blood component administration.

Stay with the patient, closely monitor and review the implemented treatment, and summon the emergency response team to help. Use the major haemorrhage protocol to alert the multidisciplinary team (including the laboratory technician) and summon help in dealing with this emergency.

Observations should be checked every 5–15 minutes in hypovolaemic shock, as they are a good indicator of improving intravascular fluid volume and restoration of tissue perfusion. BP, HR, oxygen saturation and urine output should be improving; if not, re-assess, and use the 'ABCDE' approach again. Is there any further intervention possible to help the patient? Is imaging required to help determine whether there is ongoing concealed bleeding? Does the patient need a surgical procedure to explore for and stem ongoing bleeding? Gastroenterologists should be involved if upper GI bleed is suspected. Interventional radiologists may be required to perform embolisation or other procedures to stem bleeding from the mid-GI tract or other areas that are difficult to access surgically.

REMEMBER

IVF for initial resuscitation in a patient identified as having hypovolaemic shock

Secure a large bore cannula (14G or 16G). Instigate the major haemorrhage protocol if appropriate.

Administer warm balanced crystalloids that contain sodium in the range 130–154 mmol/L (e.g. Hartmann's or Plasmalyte), with a bolus of 500 mL over 15 minutes or less. Follow with a colloid (e.g. Gelofusin or Volplex) if hypotension persists and whilst awaiting the arrival of blood to transfuse.

Do not wait for full blood count (FBC) and clotting profile results before ordering cryoprecipitate, fresh frozen plasma or platelets; ongoing bleeding depletes clotting factors, so consider replacement early in the resuscitation process.

Central venous and arterial lines can be sited to help with monitoring of the response to resuscitation. Aim for a MAP ≥65 mmHg, urine output ≥0.5 mL/kg/hr, reducing lactate levels, and if available, central venous oxygen saturation of 70%.

ABG/VBG readings can be obtained to help monitor lactate, electrolyte and haemoglobin levels and determine if acidosis is improving with resuscitation.

CONCLUSION

Overall, recognition of the critically ill or unresponsive patient should trigger prompt action to resuscitate and treat the underlying cause. Use the 'ABCDE' approach to identify the deteriorating patient and monitor for signs of improvement once resuscitation is underway. A good choice for initial fluid resuscitation is a 500 or 250 mL challenge of a balanced crystalloid. Monitor for signs of improvement; if none are apparent, consider more of the same, or an alternative such as a colloid fluid or blood components. Once the patient is stabilised, the next steps should include decisions about the location of care (general ward, high dependency unit [HDU], intensive care unit [ICU], tertiary centre), as well as whether further attempts at resuscitation should be made if the situation occurs again. These decisions should be made in conjunction with senior colleagues and the intensive care team, including discussion with the patient's family where possible.

CASE 3.1 – SEPSIS

A 32-year-old woman with no significant past medical history is admitted with a productive cough. She has right-sided basal crackles on chest auscultation.

Her observations are as follows:

HR 110 bpm (normal sinus rhythm)
BP 90/50 mmHg
RR 22 breaths/min
SpO_2 95% on room air
Temperature 38.5°C
CRT of 4 seconds

Venous blood gas (VBG):

pH 7.28
BE −8
Bicarbonate 16
Lactate 4.0
Sodium 145
Chloride 112
Potassium 4.9
Urea 9.1
Creatinine 180

What is the likely diagnosis?

The likely diagnosis in this patient is sepsis secondary to community acquired chest infection/pneumonia.

What are your priorities in treating this patient?

Address abnormalities found during the 'ABCDE' assessment.

Implement the 'Sepsis Six' – high-flow oxygen, antibiotics, IV fluid resuscitation, blood cultures, urine output and lactate measurement.

Hallmarks

Temperature >38°C or <36°C
Pulse >90 bpm
RR >20 or PaCO2 <32 mmHg
White cell count >12,000/mm^3 or <4000/mm^3
Suspected or identified source of infection

Management

Focusing on suitable fluid management in this case, a balanced crystalloid, like Hartmann's solution, would be the recommended fluid as per *Surviving Sepsis* guidelines.

Sodium chloride should be avoided because the patient is already profoundly hyperchloraemic and hyperchloraemia is linked to poor tissue perfusion and renal impairment requiring renal replacement therapy.

Of note, there is a tendency amongst junior doctors to avoid administering Hartmann's in patients with a raised lactate level. This would seem like common sense because Hartmann's in itself contains sodium lactate. However, it is important to remember that the sodium lactate component is metabolised to bicarbonate and water by the liver, thus acting as a buffer in patients with metabolic acidosis.

Lactate level is a reliable marker of tissue hypoperfusion.

Of note, this patient's potassium at 4.9 mmol/L is at the upper limit of normal. Despite Hartmann's solution containing 5 mmol/L of potassium, it is still the best option. The reason for this is that hyperchloraemia is often linked with metabolic acidosis. The body tries to compensate physiologically for the acidosis by shifting hydrogen ions into the cell in exchange for potassium which moves out of the cell into the plasma. If an alkalinising solution such as Hartmann's or Plasmalyte is administered this process gets reversed and potassium shifts back into the cell. Hence, as acidosis is reversed with appropriate fluid resuscitation, potassium will move back into the cells and the relative hyperkalaemia will correct.

Hartmann's solution should be administered as a 500-mL stat infusion since the patient is young and has no comorbidities. A more cautious initial fluid challenge of 250 mL would be recommended in frail or elderly patients or those with chronic heart failure.

The patient should constantly be reassessed for the response to the fluid challenge. The expected response in this patient to 500 mL of Hartmann's would be a drop in HR, increase in BP and an improving blood gas picture. If the response is only temporary, this suggests that there is room for more filling, whereas if sustained improvement results, then normovolaemia/euvolaemia is achieved. In this case, it would be likely that this young patient has a much greater fluid deficit in view of decompensated metabolic acidosis and would need further fluid boluses.

CASE 3.2 – ANAPHYLAXIS

A 19-year-old male attends A&E on the advice of staff at the sexual health clinic he went to first. Upon seeing the FY2 doctor, he states that he has developed a tingling sensation in the back of his throat and itching around the genital area. He has had these symptoms for about 12 hours and does not feel quite right; he has been unable to go to work. There is no significant PMH. Here is a summary of your assessment:

Airway: Patent. He is able to complete full sentences and when you inspect the throat and neck, there is no obvious abnormality. During the consultation, he starts to cough more and more violently.

Breathing: No wheeze or abnormal breath sounds auscultated. RR 22 breaths/min. Oxygen saturation 98% on air.

Circulation: Flushed appearance of the face and trunk. Cool peripheries, CRT 4 seconds. HR 100 bpm. BP 90/70 mmHg.

Disability: GCS score 15/15. Cranial and peripheral nerve examinations are normal. Capillary blood glucose level is 6.0 mmol/L. Urinalysis shows moderate leucocytes only.

Exposure: As he mentioned genital itching, an examination of the genitalia is performed. There is marked erythema and swelling around the mons pubis, scrotum and penis.

Upon further questioning, he reveals that he had sexual intercourse the previous night, and as this was with a new partner, he used a latex condom.

What is the likely diagnosis?
The likely diagnosis in this patient is mild/early stages of anaphylaxis triggered by latex condom use.

What are your priorities in treating this patient?
Measures should be taken to prevent this progressing to a severe reaction to latex. Call for help and move the patient to an area where he can be monitored for signs of deterioration, as it is not often possible to predict how quickly this can happen. The trigger has already been removed. His airway is patent; however, he is showing signs of abnormalities in breathing and circulation. Administer adrenaline (1:1000) 500 micrograms, assess if further doses are required. Administer high-flow oxygen and insert a wide-bore cannula. Although he is currently normotensive, the pulse pressure is narrow; administer a balanced crystalloid or normal saline to help maintain intravascular fluid volume. If he suddenly

becomes hypotensive, the rate of fluid administration can be sped up. He should be advised to use latex-free condoms in future.

Hallmarks

- Variable symptoms
- Exposure to a suspected or known allergen
- Acute onset of illness involving skin, mucosa or both, with respiratory or circulatory compromise (or both)

Management

The mainstay of management of anaphylaxis is to aim to prevent further clinical deterioration. Adrenaline acts as a vasopressor and is given intramuscularly at an adult dose of 0.5 mg (= 500 micrograms = 0.5 mL of 1:1000) or intravenously by a specialist at adult bolus doses of 50 micrograms = 0.5 mL of 1:10,000. An adrenaline infusion may be required. Do not delay adrenaline use, it must be administered as soon as possible after anaphylaxis has been recognised; this is why patients are given their own administration devices once the condition has been diagnosed.

Administer high-flow oxygen at 15 L/min via a non-rebreathe mask. Start IVF as soon as possible, to address hypotension and circulatory collapse. Large volumes of fluid can shift from the intravascular space into the interstitial space due to the increased permeability of capillaries. A balanced crystalloid should be given as a fluid challenge of 500 mL over 15 minutes; assess the response to this with measurement of BP, HR, RR and urine output and administer more as necessary. Use the 'ABCDE' approach to assess and manage the patient. After immediate resuscitation, administer chlorphenamine, hydrocortisone and, bronchodilators, and in specialist settings (intensive care), other vasopressors or inotropes may be used to keep the patient stable. They should remain in hospital for at least 8 hours for observation, and upon discharge, arrangements should be made for the patient to have an adrenaline auto-injector and for follow-up for investigation of other allergens.

Investigations

Baseline FBC, U&Es, clotting and liver profiles should be obtained. ABG or VBG can provide quick information about the patient's acid–base status and electrolyte abnormalities. Specifically, in anaphylaxis, mast cell tryptase levels (peak at 1–2 hours after onset) are useful in confirming anaphylaxis, especially when the diagnosis is unclear or there are concurrent conditions like asthma.

Further reading

Bunn F and Trivedi D. Colloid solutions for fluid resuscitation. *Cochrane Database Syst Rev* 2012; (6):CD001319. doi:10.1002/14651858.CD001319.pub5.

Finfer S, Bellomo R, McEvoy S, et al. Effect of baseline serum albumin concentration on outcome of resuscitation with albumin or saline in patients in intensive care units: Analysis of data from the Saline versus Albumin Fluid Evaluation (SAFE) study. *BMJ* 2006; 333: 1044–1044.

Guidet B, Martinet O, Boulain T, et al. Assessment of hemodynamic efficacy and safety of 6% hydroxyethylstarch 130/0.4 vs. 0.9% NaCl fluid replacement in patients with severe sepsis: The CRYSTMAS study. *Crit Care* 2012; 16 (3): R94. doi:10.1186/cc11358.

Maitland K, George EC, Evans JA, et al. Exploring mechanisms of excess mortality with early fluid resuscitation: Insights from the FEAST trial. *BMC Med* 2013; 11: 68. doi:10.1186/1741-7015-11-68.

Myburgh, JA and Mythen MG. Resuscitation fluids. *N Engl J Med* 2013; 369: 1243–1251. doi:10.1056/NEJMra120862.

Myburgh JA, Finter S, Bellomo R, et al. Hydroxyethyl starch or saline for fluid resuscitation in intensive care (CHEST trial group). *N Engl J Med* 2012; 367: 1901–1911. doi:10.1056/NEJMoa1209759.

NICE Guideline. *Intravenous Fluid Therapy in Adults in Hospital Guidelines.* 2013. https://www.nice.org.uk/guidance/cg174/resources/intravenous-fluid-therapy-in-over-16s-in-hospital-35109752233669.

Nolan JP and Pullinger R. Hypovolaemic shock. *BMJ* 2014; 348. doi:10.1136/bmj.g1139.

Perel P, Roberts I and Ker K. Colloids versus crystalloids for fluid resuscitation in critically ill patients. *Cochrane Database Syst Rev* 2013; (2):CD000567. doi:10.1002/14651858.CD000567.pub6.

Powell-Tuck J, Gosling P, Lobo DN, et al. *British Consensus Guidelines on Intravenous Fluid Therapy for Adult Surgical Patients.* March 2011. http://www.bapen.org.uk/pdfs/bapen_pubs/giftasup.pdf.

Raghunathan K, Murray PT, Beattie WS, et al. Choice of fluid in acute illness: What should be given? An international consensus. *BJA* 2014; 113 (5): 772–783. doi:10.1093/bja/aeu301.

Resuscitation Council UK. *Adult Advanced Life Support*. 2016. https://www.resus.org.uk/resuscitation-guidelines/adult-advanced-life-support/.

Resuscitation Council UK. *Emergency Treatment of Anaphylactic Reactions*. 2008. https://www.resus.org.uk/anaphylaxis/emergency-treatment-of-anaphylactic-reactions/.

Surviving Sepsis Campaign. *International Guidelines for Management of Severe Sepsis and Septic Shock: 2012*. http://www.sccm.org/Documents/SSC-Guidelines.pdf.

CHAPTER 4

Intravenous fluid therapy in medical patients

INTRODUCTION

The optimal fluid management of medical patients is of great importance and is often poorly managed. The role of the physician in accurately assessing fluid status, losses and requirements is critical.

Medical patients can present with multiple co-morbidities that make fluid management challenging, for example the septic patient with congestive cardiac failure (CCF).

Medical wards cannot provide the invasive monitoring and high staff to patient ratios that are found in an intensive therapy unit/high dependency unit (ITU/HDU) environment and some patients may not be appropriate for escalation to these levels of care. This means that good clinical fluid assessment, scrupulous fluid balance monitoring, and sound clinical judgement and knowledge are required by all junior doctors working on medical wards.

Decisions regarding intravenous fluid (IVF) therapy are often far from routine – do not hesitate to seek senior or specialist advice, for which this chapter is no substitute.

REMEMBER

Maintenance fluids in medical patients

'Doctor, could you just come up to the ward to write up some fluids?'

Prescribing maintenance intravenous fluids should not be considered a robotic or routine task; it is the same as prescribing medication. Careful assessment of fluid status and exacting fluid prescription is of paramount importance, as is checking the patient's most recent blood results.

When asked to prescribe maintenance fluids always consider the **reason** for IVF therapy (is it still necessary?).

Check:

- Patient fluid status
- Electrolyte requirements, recent U+Es
- Any special considerations from their medical history

Aim to encourage oral intake as much as possible.

MEDICAL CONSIDERATIONS IN FLUID ASSESSMENT AND MANAGEMENT

To cover both urine output and insensible losses, healthy adults require around 30–40 mL/kg of water over 24 hours. This equates to 2–2.5 L of fluids/day in a 70-kg adult. These requirements will be different in some groups of patients, for example those in renal failure or the frail elderly. This is discussed in detail in the sections that follow.

No fluid balance available:

- Estimated maintenance from weight
- Estimate insensible losses (0.5–1.5 L/24 hours)
- Estimate deficit: From your fluid assessment

Fluid balance available:

- Recorded intake and losses from chart
- Estimate insensible losses (0.5–1.5 L/24 hours)
- Estimate deficit: From your fluid assessment

Once the fluid requirements are known they can be written up as 500- and 1000-mL bags at the appropriate rate. Do not forget to factor in oral intake. **Where it is safe to do so**, prescribe fluids so that they will run out during the next working day so that the team looking after the patient can reassess.

Table 4.1   A guide to clinically estimating fluid deficit

Fluid deficit	Mild	Moderate	Severe
Heart rate (HR)	Normal (N)	>100	>120
Blood pressure (BP)	N	N	
		SBP < 20 mmHg decrease	SBP > 20 mmHg decrease
		DBP < 10 mmHg decrease	DBP > 10mmHg decrease
Urine output	>0.5 mg/kg/hr	<0.5 mg/kg/hr	<0.3 mg/kg/hr
% Body weight loss	3–5	5–10	10–15
Estimated deficit	<750 mL	750 mL–1.5 L	>1.5 L

REMEMBER

Ask your patient if they feel thirsty – a good sign they are not fluid depleted! However, it is important to note that elderly patients often lose their thirst awareness so in these patients it is not a good marker of fluid depletion. Also, **ensure that they have access to oral fluids and if not able to feed themselves that they are being assisted in doing so** – 10 minutes spent helping a patient drink some water is time well spent!

Typical maintenance fluid regimes in medical patients

There are a number of factors to consider when prescribing maintenance fluids in medical patients; in summary:

- '1 salt and 2 sweet': This rigid approach is completely outdated and no longer valid, as fluid therapy should be based on an individual patient's needs.

- Balanced fluids, such as Hartmann's solution and Plasmalyte, are generally the first-line choice.

- NICE guidance gives a clear approach to replacement and maintenance of fluids (see 'Further Reading' section).

- Colloids: Semi-synthetic colloids such as Geloplasma/Gelofusine are used less frequently in clinical practice. They would be a reasonable choice in patients who are thought to be in hypovolaemic cardiac arrest. They should also be considered in bleeding patients, whilst waiting for blood products to arrive.

- Blood components are the best replacement for lost blood and act as the natural colloid (see Chapter 6).

- Hypertonic solutions: Generally reserved as a 'holding measure' for patients with intracranial pathology who have evidence of raised intracranial pressure and are awaiting definitive therapy. Hypertonic saline is also used in patients with severe symptomatic hyponatraemia. Hypertonic saline should not be used outside ITU unless under direction of the endocrine team. Never give hypertonic solutions without seeking specialist, senior advice.

IVF THERAPY IN THE CONTEXT OF SPECIFIC MEDICAL PRESENTATIONS

In this section, we consider IVF therapy in the context of specific medical presentations. These have been split into the following four broad categories:

1. Fluid depletion/dehydration (for example, diarrhoea and vomiting)
2. Fluid overload (for example, CCF)
3. Complex fluid states (for example, hepatorenal syndrome [HRS])
4. Other presentations (for example, fluids at the end of life)

Fluid depletion

The management of fluid depletion is essentially to replace the fluid and electrolytes that have been lost. A large amount of fluid can be lost from the gastrointestinal (GI) tract and we have covered the basic physiology of how water and electrolytes move in and out of cells. However, one must also consider why and how fluid is depleted (Table 4.1):

a. Is my patient fluid depleted?
b. What have they had?

c. How much fluid are they taking in?

d. How much are they losing/passing as urine?

Has the patient responded to a fluid challenge?

If fluid challenge has not made a difference after what is considered an adequate amount for the patient, patient care must be escalated to a senior clinician immediately and HDU care should be considered.

Topics covered:

a. Acute kidney injury (AKI): Including rhabdomyolysis and chronic renal failure

b. Diarrhoea and vomiting

c. Burns and toxic epidermal necrolysis

d. GI bleeds: Covered in a case in Chapter 6 (see section 'Blood Components')

Fluid overload

Fluid overload is when there is too much water in the body or it has entered the wrong compartment, like excess fluid in the interstitial tissue. Management of these states is very much dependent on the origin of the fluid overload and treating the underlying cause, while ensuring symptomatic relief and off-loading the excess fluid.

Cardiac failure is one of the major causes of fluid overload and so an explanation of how cardiac failure causes fluid overload is outlined.

Topics covered:

a. CCF and pulmonary oedema

b. Liver failure and ascites

c. Chronic renal failure: Covered under AKI in fluid depleted states

Complex fluid states

In patients where complex overlapping pathology has led to fluid shifts, secondary to a variety of processes, the way ahead is rarely clear. Seek senior help early and escalate promptly to the HDU/ITU if there is not a satisfactory response to treatment. For example, consider this in cases such as the following:

a. Sepsis and CCF, chronic kidney disease (CKD)
b. AKI and CCF

These medical presentations can be very complex and each patient should be treated individually depending on the extent of each pathology. We cannot cover such complex management in a step-wise manner, and for such cases a thorough fluid assessment (outlined in Chapter 1) and senior input should be undertaken swiftly.

Electrolyte abnormalities can also cause complex fluid states as their serum concentration can be simultaneously dependent and influence the body's water content. For example, consider hyponatremia, covered in Chapter 2 in the section Electrolyte Abnormalities.

Topics covered:

a. Hepato-renal syndrome (HRS)
b. Hypercalcaemia of malignancy: Covered in Cases at the end of this chapter

Other fluid states

This includes management of conditions that are complex and do not fit into the previously mentioned categories.

Topics covered:

a. Fluids at the end of life
b. Fluids in the elderly

FLUID DEPLETION

Acute kidney injury

AKI is commonly seen in hospitalised patients. Essentially AKI encompasses acute renal deterioration of any cause.

History
Current medical problem
There are many risk factors for AKI such as the following:

- Sepsis
- Liver failure

- Heart failure (HF)
- Diabetes mellitus
- Major surgery
- Trauma
- Old age and physical frailty
- Ischaemic heart disease (IHD)
- Nephrotoxic drugs

Broadly speaking, the causes for AKI can be divided into three groups, which are as follows:

- Pre-renal
- Renal
- Post-renal

Pre-renal AKI, which is the most commonly seen type, is caused by volume depletion. Renal AKI may be caused by drugs (such as angiotensin-converting enzyme [ACE]-inhibitors) or autoimmune conditions. Post-renal AKI is caused by obstruction. It is vital to identify the cause for the AKI early, as this dictates management. It is equally important to treat the underlying condition and stop any nephrotoxic drugs.

Current fluid status

A thorough clinical assessment of the patient's volume status, as already described in Chapter 1, is of utmost importance. Patients who are deemed volume-depleted require fluid resuscitation, patients who are deemed euvolaemic do not necessarily require any IVF and patients who are clinically fluid-overloaded require loop diuretics or even emergency haemofiltration in an HDU setting (see the 'Management' section for haemofiltration criteria). The clinical aim is to achieve and maintain a euvolaemic state.

Patients with AKI can have a normal urine output (prognostically favourable), be polyuric (which tends to occur in the resolving stages of AKI) or be oligo-anuric. The latter carries the worst prognosis and managing these patients is often quite challenging, because they require very frequent assessments of their fluid status. If they are clinically euvolaemic, a 'watch and wait' strategy often has to be adopted until the patient either improves or deteriorates.

Investigations

A urine dipstick offers useful information. If more than one plus of protein is detected, send a urinary polymerase chain reaction (PCR) spot urine test. If a renal cause for the AKI is suspected, it is advisable to send a nephritic screen, complement levels, an auto-antibody screen and a myeloma screen in elderly patients. In this patient group, seek advice from a nephrologist early.

According to *NICE* Guideline 169, an urgent renal ultrasound (i.e. within 6 hours) should be performed in the following cases:

- Suspected renal obstruction
- Suspected pyonephrosis
- Patients with oligo-anuria
- Renal transplant patients

REMEMBER

If the cause of the AKI is thought to be pre-renal, patients do not necessarily require an ultrasound scan (USS) provided they are clinically improving.

Management

Treat the underlying cause

Specific management of each condition is required, which is beyond the scope of this book.

Treat the current fluid status

The *KDIGO* Guideline (2012) recommends a balanced crystalloid, such as Hartmann's or Plasmalyte, as the first-line fluid. Both fluids are alkalinising and have 'buffering' effects, which is desirable as most AKI patients frequently have a degree of metabolic acidosis and also often lose bicarbonate in the urine. Plasmalyte has the advantage that it contains less chloride than Hartmann's. There is some evidence that hyperchloraemia is an independent predictor of mortality and leads to worse patient outcomes, which is why it should be avoided.

Normal saline contains a lot of chloride (154 mmol/L) and should ideally be avoided, unless the patient has severe hyperkalaemia.

1.26% sodium bicarbonate may be an appropriate fluid to administer in AKI patients who are fluid-depleted, have a metabolic acidosis with concomitant hyperkalaemia and a low intrinsic bicarbonate level on their blood gas. It is advisable to seek senior input in these cases.

Criteria for emergency renal replacement therapy are as follows:

- Symptomatic uraemia
- Fluid overload refractory to loop diuretics, glyceryl trinitrate (GTN), morphine and continuous positive airway pressure (CPAP)/Optiflow
- A persistent severe metabolic acidosis
- Refractory severe hyperkalaemia

Review of implemented treatment

Patients with renal pathology will require regular review of their renal function via urine output and U+Es.

Special considerations – fluid management in patients with renal pathology

Fluid therapy in chronic renal failure

Clinical evaluation of volume status is vital in this patient group. Dialysis patients are usually on a fluid restriction regime and their management should always be discussed with their primary dialysis centre. The same rule applies to patients with a renal transplant. If there is clinical evidence of organ underperfusion, small aliquots of IVF may be appropriate. Balanced crystalloids should be the first-line choice. Monitor potassium and avoid hyperkalaemia.

Rhabdomyolysis

Rhabdomyolysis leads to release of myoglobin from muscle tissue. Under certain conditions, for example in volume depletion and acidic urine, myoglobin can precipitate with the body's intrinsic Tamm–Horsfall protein in the renal tubules and cause/exacerbate AKI. Early aggressive IVF therapy is the most important aspect of treatment and is required to 'flush the kidneys', increase estimated glomerular filtration rate (eGFR), minimise the nephrotoxic effects of myoglobin and aid its elimination from the body.

The treatment goal is to achieve 'high ins and outs', i.e. aggressive fluid therapy with a high urine output.

There is some evidence that urine alkalinisation may prevent precipitation of myoglobin and hence prevent AKI – pay particular attention to the urinary pH on a urine dipstick. If it is less than 6.50 (i.e. acidic), use intravenous 1.26% sodium bicarbonate to alkalinise the urine, aiming for a urinary pH of greater than 6.50. Maintain this therapy until the myoglobinuria has resolved (as evidenced by clear urine and a urine dipstick negative for blood).

Monitor the patient's U+Es, including calcium, as well as the creatine kinase (CK).

Radiological contrast and IV fluids

Patients who require investigations involving iodinated contrast agents and who either have established AKI or are at risk of contrast-induced nephropathy (same risk factors as for AKI) should have reno-protective measures instituted prior to their investigation. Unless the patient is hypervolaemic, current evidence supports intravenous pre-hydration with normal saline or 1.26% sodium bicarbonate to ensure a euvolaemic state before any contrast is administered. There is also some weak evidence that oral N-acetylcysteine may help prevent contrast-induced nephropathy.

It is advisable to familiarise yourself with your hospital's trust policy and to inform the radiology department that a patient has or is at risk of AKI. Iso- or low-osmolar agents with lower iodine contents are often selected in these cases.

You should also consider temporarily stopping any nephrotoxic drugs, particularly if the patient has significantly impaired renal function or chronic renal failure with an eGFR of less than 60 mL/min/1.73 m^2.

Post contrast exposure, the patient's renal function should be monitored for up to 5 days.

Diarrhoea and vomiting

Background physiology: GI causes of fluid depletion

Absorption and secretion of water occur throughout the intestine in normal circumstances. Diarrhoea results from disruption to the water and electrolyte transport in the small intestine. Intestinal transport mechanisms underpin the management of diarrhoea through oral fluid therapy and feeding.

A healthy adult imbibes approximately 2.5 L of fluid each day. Secretions including saliva, gastric and pancreatic juices plus bile add approximately 6.5 L. This amounts to 9 L of fluid that enter the small intestine every day.

In the small intestine, water and electrolytes are simultaneously absorbed by the villi and secreted by the epithelial crypts. Hence, there is two-way flow of water and electrolytes between the intestinal lumen and the circulation. In health, fluid absorption exceeds secretion with a net result of fluid absorption.

In normal circumstances, more than 90% of fluid is reabsorbed in the small intestine. Approximately 1 L enters the large intestine where further reabsorption takes place. Usually only 100–200 mL of water is lost in solid stools.

Decreased absorption or increased secretion in the small bowel leads to an increase in the amount of fluid entering the large bowel. When this exceeds the limited absorptive capacity of the large bowel, then diarrhoea occurs.

Absorption of water and electrolytes

- Water is absorbed down the osmotic gradient created when solutes, especially sodium, are absorbed from the gut lumen by the villous epithelial cells.
- Sodium can be absorbed directly, linked to chloride, glucose or amino acid absorption or exchanged for hydrogen ions.
- Addition of glucose to an electrolyte solution can increase sodium absorption threefold.
- Sodium is then transported out of the epithelial cells by Na^+K^+-ATPase ion pumps which transfer sodium to the extracellular fluid (ECF), increasing the osmolality.
- Water and other electrolytes then follow passively down the concentration gradient from bowel lumen through intercellular channels into the ECF.

Diarrhoea

Diarrhoea is defined by the World Health Organisation as having three or more loose or liquid stools per day, or as passing more stools than is normal for that person.

Diarrhoea is a common cause of death in the developing world. It is a relatively rare cause of death in the developed world but nevertheless left untreated and without fluid rehydration it can lead to serious morbidity. Those patients at extremes of age are at particularly high risk.

Diarrhoea types

Secretory:

- Abnormal secretion of water and electrolytes into the small bowel
- Impaired sodium absorption in the villi
- Chloride secretion continues or increases
- Net fluid secretion
- May be result of effects of bacterial toxins or viruses on bowel mucosa

Osmotic:

Presence of poorly absorbed, osmotically active substance in gut lumen causes water and salts to move rapidly across the small bowel epithelium to maintain osmotic balance.

- Can occur when lactase deficiency or glucose malabsorption is present.
- If the gut contents are hypertonic, then electrolytes and water will pass down their osmotic gradient into the gut lumen from the ECF causing diarrhoea and loss of body water.

Secretory diarrhoea is more common but intestinal infections can cause diarrhoea by both mechanisms.

Diarrhoea results in loss of water and electrolytes such as sodium, chloride, potassium and bicarbonate. There may be additional water and electrolytes lost in vomitus and through increased insensible losses due to pyrexia. These losses lead to the following:

- Dehydration (loss of water and sodium chloride)
- Metabolic acidosis due to bicarbonate loss
- Potassium depletion

Dehydration can lead to decreased blood volume (hypovolaemia), cardiovascular collapse and death if severe cases are not treated promptly. Dehydration can be classified into the following three types:

- Isotonic
- Hypertonic (hypernatraemic)
- Hypotonic (hyponatraemic)

History
Current medical problem
There are many causes of diarrhoea including the following:

- Bacterial infection, e.g. *Salmonella*, *Shigella*, *Campylobacter*, *Escherichia coli*, *Clostridium difficile*
- Viral infection, e.g. rotavirus, norovirus
- Inflammatory bowel disease
- Drugs, e.g. antibiotics, chemotherapeutic agents
- Gut ischaemia
- Appendicitis
- Food allergy/intolerance, e.g. coeliac disease

Current fluid status
Patients will generally have fluid depletion due to excess fluid loss, with varying degrees of dehydration (see 'Examination' section that follows).

Examination
Patients will be generally unwell, with nonspecific signs and symptoms of GI upset. Abdominal pain may be present, rarely with tenderness on examination. Assessment of dehydration is very important as it can cause severe morbidity.

Dehydration with 5% body weight loss
- Thirst
- Decreased skin turgor
- Tachycardia
- Dry mucous membranes/cracked lips
- Sunken eyes
- Sunken anterior fontanelle in infants
- Oliguria

Severe dehydration with 10% body weight loss
- Hypotension
- Anuria
- Cool extremities
- Reduced conscious level
- Signs of hypovolaemic shock

>10% body weight loss
- Circulatory collapse and death

Investigations
Blood tests
- Full blood count (FBC): White blood cells (WBC) may be raised, haemoglobin (Hb) might be raised in severe dehydration.
- U+Es: Hypokalaemia and hyponatraemia, urea is raised in dehydration and creatinine may be raised due to AKI caused by dehydration (pre-renal).

ECG
If electrolyte imbalance is severe, e.g. hypokalaemia-associated changes.

Stool samples
Send stool samples to isolate the causative agent.

Management
Treat the underlying cause
Patients should be isolated until the causal agent is identified and treated. Once the causal agent is treated or removed, stools usually return to normal.

Appropriate antibacterial or antiparasitic medications should be used to target the specific cause. If there is need for antibiotics, usually targeted anaerobic antibiotics guided by microbiology will be used. Some antibiotics can actually cause severe diarrhoea and colitis, such as ciprofloxacin.

Management of diarrhoeal dehydration should focus on rapidly correcting fluid and electrolyte deficits – 'rehydration therapy' – and then replacing further fluid and electrolyte loss until the diarrhoea resolves.

Fluid losses can be replaced orally or intravenously, the intravenous route usually being reserved for initial rehydration of severe cases, see the following.

Treat current fluid status

Oral rehydration therapy:

Intestinal absorption of sodium is enhanced by the active absorption of certain molecules like glucose. This glucose-linked sodium absorption can be applied to rehydrate patients using oral rehydration salt solutions. Water and other electrolytes follow sodium down the osmotic gradient and rehydration occurs. This is effective fluid replacement in most patients with secretory diarrhoea.

Oral rehydration therapy may be unsuccessful in the following:

- Patients with great stool loss, e.g. >15 mL/kg/hr
- Patients with glucose malabsorption
- Patients with severe unrelenting vomiting

In cases of severe dehydration where life is endangered, initial rehydration must be achieved rapidly and this requires intravenous infusion of water and electrolytes. The intravenous route is also warranted where patients are unable to drink or have paralytic ileus.

IVF can rapidly restore blood volume and correct shock. A number of IVF are available but all are deficient in some of the electrolytes required to restore the deficits caused by acute diarrhoeal dehydration. Even where intravenous rehydration is required in the initial treatment of dehydration, oral fluid replacement should be co-instituted at the earliest opportunity.

IVF rehydration therapy:

There are many intravenous solutions available and in extreme situations; even intravenous coconut water has been successfully utilised!

Hartmann's solution, also known as Ringer's lactate solution, is the best readily available IVF option. Hartmann's is isotonic with blood and contains 130 mmol/L of sodium and 28 mmol/L lactate, which is metabolised to bicarbonate that can correct acidosis. Hartmann's contains no glucose and only low concentrations of potassium but these can be provided through additional intake of oral rehydration salts when appropriate. Hartmann's solution can be used universally to correct dehydration secondary to diarrhoea and in all patient age groups.

It should be noted that 5% plain dextrose solution is not a suitable intravenous solution as it does not contain any electrolytes, correct acidosis or effectively treat hypovolaemia.

Review of the implemented treatment

Treatment should be reviewed after implementation; monitor the patient closely for warning signs of fluid overload or continued dehydration. Special attention to electrolytes is needed to ensure the losses have been replaced and normal values are not exceeded. Thus, all patients receiving electrolyte replacement therapy need regular serial blood tests.

Special considerations

The following guideline should be considered when treating children:

* Diarrhoea and vomiting caused by gastroenteritis in under-fives: diagnosis and management *NICE* guidelines [CG84], published date: April 2009

Vomiting

Vomiting is a reflex action where stomach contents are forcefully ejected through the mouth. It is mediated by the vomiting centre, which resides centrally in the reticular formation of the medulla and receives impulses from the chemoreceptor trigger zone, heart, GI tract, abdominal organs and peritoneum via sympathetic nerves and the vagus nerve. The act of vomiting is coordinated via motor impulses though the cranial nerves to the upper GI tract and through spinal nerves to the abdominal muscles and diaphragm.

History

Current medical problem

There are many causes of prolonged vomiting such as the following:

* Chemotherapy-related
* Drug-related, e.g. opiates, antibiotics
* Infection-related/gastroenteritis: viral or bacterial
* Pyloric stenosis
* Small bowel obstruction
* Mesenteric ischaemia
* Pancreatitis
* Raised intracranial pressure, e.g. brain tumour
* Poisoning
* Pregnancy: Hyperemesis gravidarum

GI causes:

- Gastroenteritis, bacterial or viral
- Gastritis
- Food poisoning
- Gastroesophageal reflux disease (GORD)
- Pyloric stenosis
- Bowel obstruction
- Peritonitis
- Paralytic ileus
- Pancreatitis

Drugs:

- Opiates/opioids
- Chemotherapeutic agents
- Antibiotics

Central nervous system causes:

- Ménière's disease
- Concussion
- Migraine
- Brain tumours
- Benign intracranial hypertension and hydrocephalus

Metabolic causes:

- Hypercalcaemia
- Uraemia
- Adrenal insufficiency
- Hypo/hyperglycaemia

Pregnancy:

- Hyperemesis gravidarum

Current fluid status

Prolonged vomiting can result in dehydration and potential electrolyte imbalance. Vomiting of gastric contents leads to direct hydrochloric acid loss (protons/H$^+$ and chloride ions/Cl$^-$). Parietal cells in the stomach produce more hydrochloric acid (HCl) and in doing so they secrete bicarbonate ions into the bloodstream. This occurrence is known as the alkaline tide. This increases the blood pH. Combined, this results in hypochloraemic metabolic alkalosis (low chloride and high bicarbonate levels with a raised blood pH). Hypokalaemia and hyponatraemia may also be present.

Examination and investigation

Dehydration in vomiting will present in the same way as in diarrhoea; see the aforementioned section for signs, symptoms and investigations of dehydration.

Management

Treat underlying cause

- The underlying cause and duration of vomiting should be elucidated and treated.
- The sequelae and complications of nausea and vomiting (e.g. fluid depletion, hypokalaemia, and metabolic alkalosis) should be identified and corrected.
- Targeted treatment should be provided, when possible (e.g. surgery for bowel obstruction).

Treat current fluid status

The fluid replacement treatment of dehydration secondary to prolonged vomiting begins with an assessment of the extent of dehydration and measurement of serum electrolytes. These findings will guide the required fluid management.

In less severe cases, rehydration can still be achieved via the oral route with oral rehydration salt solutions.

The classical cause of hypochloraemic metabolic alkalosis is pyloric stenosis in infants. It should be noted that this is classified as a medical as opposed to a surgical emergency and it is essential that fluid and electrolyte loss be corrected prior to any operation proceeding. In these cases, initial replacement is with 0.9% normal saline along with dextrose and subsequently, potassium supplementation.

Successful fluid resuscitation has been achieved when the patient is well perfused and serum electrolytes have returned to normal values with particular attention paid to chloride and bicarbonate levels.

Review of the implemented treatment
Same as for diarrhoea, as mentioned previously.

Burns

History
Current medical problem
Burns or adverse drug reactions such as toxic epidermal necrolysis (TEN). It is important that the 24-hour period be determined as commencing from the time of the burn and not the time of presentation.

Current fluid status
Burns can result in massive fluid loss as the skin usually acts as a barrier without which intracellular and interstitial fluid can evaporate. Thus, patients suffering with burns will usually exhibit fluid depletion.

Examination
An assessment of burn surface area (BSA) can be made using the rule of nines and is carried out with the patient fully exposed. Care should be taken to minimise exposure time during assessment as burns patients can become hypothermic very quickly.

The rule of nines divides the body into areas which are given a percentage of total body surface. The following body areas are presumed to account for 9% of BSA each: head, arm, chest and abdomen. The following body areas are presumed to account for 18% of BSA each: back and leg. Calculation of total BSA can be made by estimating the extent of burns across different body parts and then adding them together.

Most emergency departments will also have a Lund–Browder chart which can be used to make a quick assessment of burn area.

The most commonly used formula in the United Kingdom to predict total fluid requirement (in the first 24 hours) is the Parkland formula (see 'Management' section).

Investigations
Bloods

- FBC: ↑Hb due to fluid depletion and Hb concentration
- U+Es: ↑K released from damaged cells. ↑Creatinine, ↑urea caused by pre-renal AKI in cases of insufficient fluid resuscitation
- Arterial blood gas (ABG): ↑lactate, ↑base excess and metabolic acidosis due to hypovolaemia and hypoperfusion

Management
Treat the underlying cause
Management of burns is a specialist subject and will not be covered here. Essentially, it consists of ensuring the burns remain clean and no suprainfection develops, minimising heat loss and allowing healing to develop. A large amount of fluid can be lost through burns and appropriate fluid management is crucial.

Treat the current fluid status
Fluid management in burns rests on initial resuscitation and subsequent calculation of replacement fluids based on the patient's percentage burn surface area (BSA).

The Parkland formula can be used, where total replacement fluid is a product of weight and BSA multiplied by 4 mL (fluid required in 24 hours = BSA × weight [kg] × 4 mL).

Resuscitation should involve rapid clinical assessment of the patient's fluid status including blood pressure (BP), heart rate (HR) and capillary refill time (CRT). Be sure to assess both injured and non-injured limbs since the burn itself can affect assessment of perfusion.

Large bore intravenous access should be inserted and resuscitation commenced with warmed Hartmann's solution. The presence of shock necessitates a search for another cause (trauma or bleeding) since significant hypovolaemia is unlikely to be due to the burn injury alone.

A urinary catheter should be inserted aiming for a urine output of at least 0.5 mL/kg/hr in adults and 1 mL/kg/hr in children. If this is not achieved then resuscitation fluids should be increased.

Once the total fluid requirement for the first 24 hours has been calculated, any fluid that has already been administered should be subtracted from this amount.

The remaining volume should then be divided in half. This is the amount that should be delivered within the first 8 hours; the remainder should be given over the following 16 hours.

Review of the implemented treatment
It is important to re-assess your patient frequently to judge the adequacy of resuscitation. Accurate fluid assessment may not be possible due to insensible losses from the burns area, therefore base your

assessment on other signs and symptoms that might indicate fluid depletion: thirst, cardiovascular parameters, urine output.

Special considerations

Hypovolaemia is rarely due to the burn alone. Be sure to look for other sources of blood loss or trauma.

Guidelines

- Review the Parkland diagram for assessment of burns.

Electrolytes

- Regular monitoring of electrolytes is needed as both water and salts are lost from the burns.

FLUID OVERLOAD

Background physiology: Cardiology causes for fluid overload

Management of fluid status in patients with cardiovascular disease must take into account the extent of underlying disease and the immediate management of life-threatening conditions. Use the ABCDE method (see Chapter 3), addressing any emergency situations first.

Background

Cardiac failure arises when the heart's work as a pump becomes inadequate in supplying the cell's metabolic requirements. There are many causes of heart failure (HF), ischeamic heart disease (IHD) being the most common one, resulting in decreased cardiac output. Cardiac output is influenced by: preload (volume of blood going into the right side of the heart), afterload (pressure against which the left side of the heart contracts), myocardial contractility and HR.

Here are some examples:

- Myocardial infarction (MI) will cause a decrease in contractility due to infarcted myocardium being replaced by inflexible scar tissue.
- Hypertension (HTN) will lead to an increase in systemic vascular resistance, resulting in increased work of the heart.
- Valvular disease: aortic stenosis increases afterload, whereas aortic regurgitation increases preload.
- Conduction problems, such as arrhythmias and heart blocks, affect HR.

Congestive cardiac failure

This condition describes failure of both the right and left sides of the heart, often as a result of failure of one side eventually impacting on the other. The heart pumps inadequately so that excess fluid accumulates in the vascular tree, which eventually seeps out into the interstitium and causes oedema.

> **REMEMBER**
>
> Mean Arterial Pressure = Cardiac Output × Systemic Vascular Resistance
> Cardiac Output = HR × Stroke Volume

Decreased cardiac output will in turn trigger:

- Increased autonomic sympathetic activity.
- The alpha-1 receptors will increase peripheral vasoconstriction and reduce venous compliance, leading to a rise in systemic vascular resistance.
- The beta receptors will increase cardiac rate and contractility, which will put more strain on the heart.
- The Renin–angiotensin–aldosterone system (RAAS) is activated and increases the sodium and water content of the body, increasing the blood volume, leading to a rise in both preload and afterload.
- ADH levels rise, causing water retention which increases the blood volume and preload.

The body's response to HF is the same as in massive haemorrhage, and results in increased blood volume, afterload, preload, cardiac rate and contractility, which in turn worsens the HF.

History
Current fluid status
Symptoms of left ventricular failure:

- Shortness of breath (SOB), orthopnoea, paroxysmal nocturnal dyspnoea (PND), cough (pink frothy sputum), nocturia, tiredness, weakness.

Symptoms of right ventricular failure:

- Increasing leg swelling, increasing abdominal girth, nausea, anorexia.

Current fluid status

- Increased extracellular fluid volume (ECFV): Fluid overload.

Sodium content

- Normal: increased sodium = increased water (so this is a sodium regulation problem, e.g. RAAS).
- Reduced (hyponatraemia): increased sodium < increased water (so this is a water and sodium regulation problem, e.g. inappropriate ADH activation).

Tonicity

- Increased due to raised sodium levels
- Increased due to glucose in hyperglycaemia, diabetic ketoacidosis (DKA)

Past medical history

Possible cardiovascular disease: MI, angina, atrial fibrillation (AF), CCF, CKD, HTN.

Medication

- Anti-hypertensives
- Diuretics
- Beta-blockers
- ACE inhibitors
- Electrolyte supplement

Examination

Signs of left ventricular failure:

- Any signs of fluid in the lungs: third and fourth heart sounds, tachycardia, tachypnoea, wheeze, increased respiratory rate, cold peripheries, muscle wasting.

Signs of right ventricular failure:

- Any sign of excess fluid in the periphery: peripheral/sacral oedema, ascites, facial engorgement, raised jugular venous pressure (JVP).

Investigations

Bloods

- FBC: ↓Hb will put extra strain on the heart.
- U+Es: ↑creatinine, ↑urea, ↑K due to diuretics, CKD, AKI

- Liver profile: ↑alanine aminotransferase (ALT) + alkaline phosphatase (ALP) in right-sided failure indicates hepatic congestion. ↓Albumin (oedema)
- Cardiac enzymes: Troponin to assess for MI, brain natriuretic peptide (BNP) is the biomarker of HF; >100 ng/L is diagnostic.
- ABG: Respiratory failure due to pulmonary oedema, acidosis due to renal failure or ↑K, raised anion gap due to secondary causes such as hyperglycaemia or alcohol.

ECG
AF, ischaemia, MI new/old, conduction abnormality, dysrhythmias.

Imaging
- Chest radiograph: Signs of fluid overload: cardiomegaly, upper lobe diversion, alveolar oedema, interstitial oedema and pleural effusion.
- Echocardiogram: An ejection fraction (EF) of less than 54% indicates left ventricular systolic failure but note that EF can be greater than 54% in diastolic failure, where the essential problem is 'stiffness' of the heart muscle.
- Ultrasound: Right-sided HF can be indicated by cardiac cirrhosis/ free fluid around the liver and congested hepatic veins. Inferior vena cava assessment can also give information about the systemic vascular resistance and preload.

Management
In this situation, it is important to optimise the patient's preload, without exacerbating fluid overload (remember the Frank–Starling mechanism). Cautious small fluid boluses, generally with a balanced crystalloid, should be delivered if the patient is deemed volume-deplete. Endpoints of resuscitation, such as BP, HR and urine output response, should be reviewed 10–15 minutes after administration of a fluid challenge.

Fluid: These patients will not usually require supplementation with IV fluids, but if IV fluids are needed, use ***a balanced crystalloid.***

Treat the underlying cause
- Manage underlying cause of HF, e.g. valve disease, dysrhythmias, ischaemia.

- Manage exacerbating factors: infection, anaemia, HTN, thyroid disease.
- Medication review: nonsteroidal anti-inflammatory drugs (NSAIDs) contribute to fluid retention, verapamil is negatively ionotropic, beta-blockers, although indicated in chronic HF, can exacerbate acute CCF. Consider omitting other anti-hypertensives if diuretics or a GTN-infusion will be used.

Treat fluid overload
Acute pulmonary oedema

- 100% oxygen via a non-rebreathe mask.
- Furosemide 20–120-mg IV stat (depending on the patient's body size, larger patients need more diuretic).
- GTN spray two puffs sublingually, if no improvement and SBP >90 mmHg, consider starting a GTN infusion.
- Morphine 2.5–10-mg IV slowly (dose depends on the patient's body size).
- Patients may require non-invasive ventilation (NIV)/CPAP if they are not responding to the aforementioned measures.
- Diuretic therapy can be helpful, but remember to review the patient's sodium and potassium levels before initiating.

Special considerations
Differential diagnoses
Chronic obstructive pulmonary disease (COPD), pulmonary embolism (PE).

Guidelines
- Framingham criteria for CCF.
- New York Health Association classification of HF.
- *NICE guideline 108 for the treatment of chronic CCF:* Use of ACE inhibitors, beta-blockers, mineralocorticoid receptor agonists such as Spironolactone or Eplerenone, digoxin, vasodilators such as a nitrate, hydralazine or calcium-channel blocker. More specialised treatments for HF include ultrafiltration (in diuretic-resistance), device therapy (biventricular pacing and ventricular assist devices) and heart transplantation.

REMEMBER

Furosemide is a loop diuretic; it can cause hypokalaemia and hypernatraemia, by way of its action on the Na/K/ CL co-transporter pump system in the ascending limb of nephrons. Patients on diuretics require regular monitoring of their U+Es.

Review treatment

- Patients will require regular/continuous monitoring (BP, ECG, saturations) until they are stabilised; consider HDU care.
- Patients with decompensated HF and AKI will often require invasive haemodynamic monitoring and therefore HDU care. Getting the fluid balance right in this particular group of patients is one of the most challenging situations to be encountered in medicine!
- Continuous BP monitoring, titrate GTN to ensure systolic BP >100 mmHg.
- Urine output monitoring, strict fluid balance chart. Patients will often require fluid restriction.
- Dietary sodium restriction.
- Daily weights, as changes will represent fluid level alteration.
- Repeat U+Es with diuretic use to ensure there is no evolving electrolyte abnormality or worsening renal function.
- Serial ECGs.
- Rate-control if the patient is in fast AF. Digoxin is the drug of choice in this situation. Beta-blockers should be avoided/temporarily discontinued in acute HF.
- If the patient is tachypnoeic or saturations are <90% despite high-flow oxygen consider NIV, CPAP or Optiflow. Senior support is required.
- If the patient becomes shocked and systolic BP <85 mmHg consider vasoactive support with continuous ECG and BP monitoring, senior support and HDU care are required.
- If the acute HF develops in the context of an acute coronary syndrome, percutaneous coronary intervention may be required urgently. Discuss with a tertiary centre.

Liver disease

Chronic liver disease and cirrhosis

Cirrhosis is the condition where healthy liver cells are replaced by scar tissue and one of its most common complications is ascites (the accumulation of fluid in the peritoneal cavity).

Ascites

It is thought that peripheral arterial vasodilatation leads to an under-filled circulatory system, thereby activating the RAAS via its baro-receptors. This leads to sympathetic nervous system (SNS) and non-osmotic release of antidiuretic hormone (ADH) and results in sodium and water retention. As the liver disease worsens this results in fluid retention and ascites.

Hepatorenal syndrome

This is a type of functional renal failure due to low cardiac output and poor renal perfusion. It is managed using drugs that restore renal blood flow through peripheral arterial vasoconstriction, renal vasodilatation and plasma volume expansion (see more detail in the section 'Complex Fluid States').

History

Current medical problem

Patients with liver disease can present either with acute liver failure (see 'Special Considerations' section that follows) or as exacerbation of chronic liver disease either in compensated or decompensated state. The worsening hepatic function could be the natural progression of liver disease or due to another concurrent medical problem. Liver disease is very complex and it is beyond the scope of this book to cover the aetiology and management of liver disease.

The following sections on History, Examination, Investigation and Management are also applicable for the HRS Syndrome section and are repeated in that section with specific focus on HRS.

Current fluid status

Ask about the acute presentation; ask in particular about the following:

- Duration of any symptoms
- Nausea, vomiting, fatigue, weakness

- Decreased urine production
- Jaundice with dark urine
- Symptoms of ascites: Abdominal swelling, dyspnoea
- Symptoms of bacterial peritonitis: Signs of infection with abdominal pain/tenderness with ascites
- Confusion and altered sleep/wake cycle (symptoms of hepatic encephalopathy)

Past medical history
- Known chronic liver disease.
- Current or recent viral or alcoholic hepatitis.
- Past episodes of ascites/spontaneous bacterial peritonitis.
- Family history of liver problems.
- Alcohol: Ask about alcohol intake, current and historical. In particular, are they currently abstinent and if so, for how long?

Examination

Assess for signs of chronic liver disease such as palmar erythema, spider naevi, caput medusae, altered pattern of body hair ('hairless man'), gynaecomastia and decompensation (jaundice, ascites).

Check for a liver flap (asterixis) and confusion which are suggestive of encephalopathy.

Fluid status
- Assessing fluid status in patients with ascites can be challenging. Remember that these patients can be intravascularly deplete.
- Pay particular attention to the JVP; check CRT and monitor the urine output to assess this.
- They may also have fluid overload due to renal dysfunction and/or excess IV fluid therapy.

Investigations

All patients with acute liver failure and ascites need an urgent ascitic tap to rule out spontaneous bacterial peritonitis

Bloods

- FBC: Macrocytic anaemia.
- U+Es: Creatinine can be elevated, sodium <130 mmol/L suggests HRS.
- Clotting: Be aware that while many liver patients will have deranged clotting screens, they are in fact in a coagulopathic state so may require thromboprophylaxis.
- Liver function tests (LFTs): A full liver screen should be carried out if the aetiology of the liver disease is not known.
- Serum lactate (levels over 3 mmol/L signify poor prognosis).
- Blood glucose at least 2–hourly.

Sepsis is a common precipitant of decompensated chronic liver disease so ensure a full septic screen is sent.

Imaging

- Abdominal USS with portal and hepatic vein Dopplers to look at liver architecture and look for signs of portal HTN/thrombus and also to characterise small volume ascites.
- Chest x-ray (CXR) may show raised diaphragm (splinting from ascites).

Fluid assessment

- Urinary catheter
- Consider use of a cardiac output monitor

Management
Treat underlying cause

Supportive therapy whilst liver function recovers: Ensure bowels opened at least twice a day to prevent encephalopathy, give lactulose to promote NH_4 excretion in the bowel and ensure adequate nutritional support.

Ascitic drains (with IV albumin cover to prevent post-paracentesis circulatory problems) will reduce discomfort in tense ascites. Shunt placement can also be considered in order to redistribute fluid.

The definitive treatment is a liver transplant, where indicated.

Treat the current fluid status

Restricting water intake:
ADH release results in water retention and consequent dilutional hyponatraemia. However, there is no evidence that water restriction in cirrhotic patients improves hyponatraemia.

Sodium restriction:
This is often done through dietary restriction.

Diuretics:
Spironolactone is commonly used and has been shown to be more efficacious than salt restriction alone.

Review of the implemented treatment
Patients with liver disease need frequent review as their fluid status can fluctuate.

Special considerations
Acute liver disease
Patients with abnormal LFTs and coagulopathy should ideally be admitted to an HDU for close monitoring.

These patients may require significant fluid resuscitation in the acute period. There is often a tendency by practitioners to avoid sodium-containing fluid (as per the management of chronic liver disease) but in these patients this can often lead to cerebral oedema and subsequent seizures. Vasoactive support may also be required.

COMPLEX FLUID STATES

Hepato-renal syndrome
HRS is a state of renal failure and fluid shifts in the context of advanced liver disease. It occurs in about 4% of patients with decompensated cirrhosis, and in about 30% of patients with cirrhosis and spontaneous bacterial peritonitis.

It is thought to be caused by a severe reduction in renal perfusion, the pathogenesis of which is not fully understood but is likely a result of a combination of the following:

- Splanchnic vasodilatation reducing the effective arterial blood volume and thus MAP and renal perfusion

- Over-activation of the RAS and synthesis of vasoactive mediators causing renal vasoconstriction affecting both renal perfusion and glomerular microcirculatory dynamics
- Impaired cardiac function due to cirrhotic cardiomyopathy.

There are two types of HRS:

Type 1: Characterised by a rapid decline in renal function (a doubling of serum creatinine in less than 2 weeks), which is usually triggered by a precipitating event such as infection or an alcoholic hepatitis precipitating decompensation of liver disease. It is usually associated with a coagulopathy and marked jaundice.

Type 2: This is a steady and progressive decline in renal function which is associated with refractory ascites and sodium retention (due to a dysfunctional renin–angiotensin system in chronic liver disease).

History
Current medical problem
There is no one specific test that can establish HRS. The major diagnostic criteria (all of which must be present) are as follows:

- Advanced acute or chronic liver disease with failure
- Raised serum creatinine (typically >200 μmol/L), or reduced creatinine clearance
- No sustained improvement with fluid resuscitation
- Proteinuria <0.5 g/day
- Normal renal tract ultrasound
- Other causes of renal impairment excluded (e.g. hypovolaemia, sepsis, membranous glomerulonephritis [which could be secondary to hepatitis B]), renal tubular abnormalities, obstruction, use of radio-contrast agents

Type 1 HRS and severe type 2 HRS are serious, life-threatening conditions. Seek senior advice and get specialist input early.

Current fluid status
Ask about the acute presentation, the following in particular:

- Duration of any symptoms
- Nausea, vomiting, fatigue, weakness

- Decreased urine production
- Jaundice with dark urine
- Symptoms of ascites: Abdominal swelling, dyspnoea
- Symptoms of bacterial peritonitis: Signs of infection with abdominal pain/tenderness with ascites
- Confusion and altered sleep/wake cycle (symptoms of hepatic encephalopathy)

Past medical history
- Known chronic liver disease.
- Current or recent viral or alcoholic hepatitis.
- Past episodes of ascites/spontaneous bacterial peritonitis.
- Family history of liver/kidney problems.
- *Alcohol:* ask about alcohol intake, current and historical. In particular, are they currently abstinent and if so, for how long?

Medications
Ask about and check the chart for any nephrotoxic agents such as the following:

- Aminoglycoside antibiotics
- NSAIDs
- Antiviral agents (e.g. interferon in Hepatitis C)
- Diuretics
- ACE inhibitors and angiotensin blockers

Examination
Patients will typically have a low BP and bounding pulse. Look for signs of chronic liver disease such as palmar erythema, spider naevi, caput medusae, altered pattern of body hair ('hairless man'), gynaecomastia and decompensation (jaundice, ascites).

Check for a liver flap (asterixis) and confusion which are suggestive of encephalopathy.

Fluid status
- Assessing fluid status in patients with ascites can be challenging. Remember that these patients can be intravascularly depleted.

- Pay particular attention to the JVP; check CRT and monitor the urine output to assess this.
- They may also have fluid overload due to renal dysfunction and/or excess IV fluid therapy.

Investigations

All patients with acute liver failure and ascites need an urgent ascitic tap to rule out spontaneous bacterial peritonitis.

Bloods

- Bloods including FBC, U+Es, LFTs and clotting.
- Creatinine will be elevated.
- Sodium <130 mmol/L suggests HRS.
- Be aware that while many liver patients will have deranged clotting screens, they are in fact in a coagulopathic state so may require thromboprophylaxis.

Sepsis is a common precipitant of decompensated chronic liver disease so ensure a full septic screen is sent.

- A full liver screen should be carried out if the aetiology of the liver disease is not known.

Urine dipstick: testing for proteinuria and haematuria – marked proteinuria and haematuria indicate renal parenchymal disease rather than HRS. Renal biopsy may be required if HRS is still strongly suspected in these cases.

Imaging

- Renal USS to rule out obstruction
- Abdominal USS with portal and hepatic vein Dopplers to look at liver architecture and look for signs of portal HTN/thrombus and also to characterise small volume ascites
- CXR may show raised diaphragm (splinting from ascites)

Management

Treat underlying cause

- HRS will rarely recover unless liver function does: The goal of treatment is to support the liver and perfuse the kidneys.

- Supportive therapy whilst liver function recovers: Ensure bowels opened at least twice a day to prevent encephalopathy, give lactulose to promote NH_4 excretion in the bowel and ensure adequate nutritional support.
- Ascitic drains (with IV albumin cover to prevent post-paracentesis circulatory problems) will reduce discomfort in tense ascites.
- Stop nephrotoxic drugs including diuretics.
- The definitive treatment is a liver transplant, where indicated.

Treat current fluid status
- Hypovolaemia requires correction with crystalloids/albumin or blood products. Albumin may have specific immunomodulatory effects.
- Once the patient is euvolaemic, fluid restriction to 1–1.5 L/day should be instituted to prevent dilutional hyponatraemia.

Review treatment
- Fluid balance must be scrupulously monitored and these patients require daily blood tests.
- Have a low threshold for ITU referral. These patients may require haemodynamic monitoring and vasoactive support to maintain perfusion.
- If they are not improving then they may need haemodialysis or filtration while liver function recovers, or as a bridge to transplant.
- Transjugular intrahepatic portosystemic shunt (TIPSS) has been shown in some small studies to have short-term benefits.

Special considerations

A variety of other treatments including N-acetylcysteine, misoprostol and ACE inhibitors have not been shown to have any benefit in HRS.

Electrolytes

Remember hyponatraemia is common and may be exacerbated by overzealous use of IVFs. Hyperkalaemia in HRS may be refractory to treatment and require dialysis.

OTHER IMPORTANT PRESENTATIONS

Fluids at the end of life

This is a difficult issue, and one that causes much heartache for relatives and health care teams alike. Seek advice from your palliative care teams. One of the main concerns raised by relatives of dying patients about the Liverpool Care Pathway was early withdrawal of nutrition and IVF. Hence, new guidance of the Leadership Alliance for Care of Dying People suggests continuing both unless the patient is deemed to be imminently dying.

Siting IV cannulas in dying patients can be challenging and the data shows little benefit for fluids at the end of life. In these cases, it is often appropriate to administer fluids subcutaneously via a butterfly syringe, usually a litre of saline over 24 hours.

Fluids in elderly patients

The principles of fluid therapy in older patients remains the same as in all patients; however, there are a few considerations to be borne in mind.

In particular, a low oral intake or swallowing difficulties are not an indication for IV fluid replacement, with all the attendant risks. Has the patient been assessed by dieticians and a speech and language therapist? What is the long-term plan for nutrition and hydration?

These patients may well have a degree of cardiac or renal impairment and this may not be formally diagnosed, so care is required when prescribing fluids – do not give large volumes without rechecking the patient's fluid status.

Older, frail patients may have a low body weight and fluids should be prescribed appropriately. Three litres of saline in 24 hours in a 40-kg patient is probably not beneficial!

A chronic low-grade hyponatraemia is relatively common in the elderly. Do not be tempted to over-investigate.

CONCLUSION

In this chapter, we have covered the fluid management of common medical presentations by dividing them according to the pathological fluid status they would cause. We have outlined the common causes, specific examinations and investigation findings that you should focus on. The 'Management' section was divided into general treatment (which, at most, consists only of an outline) and specific fluid management. For full medical management of the conditions, as mentioned before, please seek senior help and other core medical texts (for examples see the 'Further Reading' section). We hope that the 'Fluid Management' sections have highlighted the approach to fluid prescribing and management and have armed you with tools to select the appropriate IVF, with particular attention to matching the electrolyte content of the IVF, for specific medical conditions.

The scope of this book is finite and we have focused on the common medical conditions. We have not covered all possible topics, such as endocrine pathologies (apart from diabetes mellitus in a case about DKA). We hope the examples covered here will provide you with the tools to adequately assess and treat your patients.

Developing a good knowledge and understanding of fluid therapies is crucial to becoming a skilled physician. Always consider your plans for fluid management carefully and take every opportunity to learn from complex cases.

CASE 4.1 – RE-FEEDING SYNDROME

A 45-year-old cachectic man with a history of alcohol excess was admitted with seizures. The patient is being treated for alcohol withdrawal and commenced on a regime of chlordiazepoxide, multivitamins and energy drinks by the ward doctor.

After 2 days, blood tests show hypophosphataemia, hypokalaemia and hypomagnesaemia.

What is the likely diagnosis?

Re-feeding syndrome

Re-feeding syndrome was initially discovered in Japanese prisoners of war after World War II. After a prolonged period of malnutrition the body's main energy source becomes ketone bodies rather than glucose/carbohydrates and the body becomes depleted in macro- and micronutrients, including electrolytes. Initiation of sudden and full enteral or parenteral nutrition leads to an increase in metabolic rate and switch back to glucose-based metabolism, with an increase of insulin secretion.

This anabolic state and increased insulin levels result in an increased need for phosphate (required for ATP synthesis). This results in fluid and electrolyte shifts.

Hallmarks of the syndrome are as follows:

- Hypophosphataemia
- Hypomagnesaemia
- Vitamin deficiencies
- Hypokalaemia
- Volume overload

Management

- The dietitian should review the patient daily. They normally recommend a slow build-up to the full caloric requirements over a few days.
- Daily monitoring of U+Es, including phosphate and magnesium.
- Replace electrolytes (enterally and IV).
- If the patient is showing signs and symptoms of re-feeding syndrome: Slow the rate of feeding, check U+Es regularly, replace electrolyte deficiencies, involve a dietitian, review for signs of fluid overload.

CASE 4.2 – HYPERCALCAEMIA

An 82-year-old man with known prostate cancer is admitted to hospital with lower back pain, constipation and confusion. His blood tests show the following:

Urea 20 mmol/L
Creatinine 120 mmol/L
Potassium 4.5 mmol/L
Calcium 3.8 mmol/L

What is the main abnormality and what is the most likely underlying diagnosis?

Hypercalcaemia

- In this particular case, the patient's severe hypercalcaemia is most likely secondary to bony metastases.
- Generally, the two most common causes of hypercalcaemia are primary hyperparathyroidism and malignancy.

CASE 4.2 – HYPERCALCAEMIA (continued)

Hallmarks
- 'Stones, bones, abdominal groans and psychic moans'
- Renal: nephrogenic diabetes insipidus
- GI tract: constipation, pancreatitis, nausea, anorexia
- Psychiatric: confusion, agitation, depression

Investigations
- Back imaging (lumbar x-ray/CT/MRI)
- Prostate-specific antigen (PSA)

Management
The most important part of the management is aggressive re-hydration with Plasmalyte or normal saline. Hartmann's solution can also be used but be aware that it contains 2 mmol/L of calcium. Make sure there is an accurate fluid chart available. Consider a bisphosphonate like Pamidronate, but only once the patient is clinically euvolaemic. Treat the underlying cause and consider referral to a specialist team, in this case oncology, for consideration of radiotherapy ± anti-hormonal treatment.

CASE 4.3 – DIABETIAC KETOACIDOSIS

A 28-year-old man with known type 1 diabetes mellitus presents with a 2-day history of gastroenteritis. The patient appears very unwell, tachypnoeic RR 40 breaths/min, BP 95/45 mmHg, HR 110 beats/min, CRT 5 seconds.

What is the most likely underlying diagnosis?

Diabetic ketoacidosis
Hallmarks of the syndrome are:

1. Acidosis: venous pH <7.3 OR bicarbonate <15 mmol/L
2. Hyperglycaemia: capillary glucose >11 mmol/L
3. Presence of ketones: capillary ketones >3 mmol/L OR urine ketones minimum ++

Management
General management of DKA according to the Joint British Diabetes Societies Inpatient Care Group:

- Immediate management: Start normal saline with potassium.
- Fixed rate intravenous insulin infusion (FRIII) after IVF has been commenced. Correct blood glucose slowly at a rate

not exceeding 3 mmol/L/hr to avoid large osmotic shifts (see Chapter 2).

- FRIII is 50 units actrapid insulin in 50-mL normal saline delivered at 0.1 units/kg/hr (equivalent to 0.1 mL/kg/hr)
- The aim is to clear the blood of ketones, aiming for a fall in blood ketone levels of at least 0.5 mmol/hr.
- Particular attention should be paid to potassium levels which should be kept within normal range (no potassium replacement in IVF, only for serum values of potassium >5.5 mmol/L).
- Hypoglycaemia should be avoided.

Fluid management

Normal saline with premixed potassium is recommended on the ward (as per *National Prescribing Service* guidelines), as per national guidelines for treatment of DKA. In a high-dependency setting, Hartmann's solution is often used. There is currently no convincing evidence suggesting that normal saline is superior to Hartmann's in these patients. The main advantage of normal saline is that potassium can easily be added. As the acidosis corrects, shifts of potassium will occur. In most hospitals, these patients are looked after in a high-dependency setting which allows close monitoring of vital signs, fluid balance and electrolytes.

Further reading

Campbell-Falck D, Thomas T, Falck TM, Tutuo N, and Clem K. The intravenous use of coconut water. *Am J Emerg Med* 2000; 18 (1): 108.

Dellinger RP, Levy MM, Rhodes A, et al. Surviving sepsis campaign: International guidelines for management of severe sepsis and septic shock: 2012. *Crit Care Med* 2013; 41 (2): 580–637. doi:10.1097/CCM.0b013e31827e83af.

For management of DKA: https://www.bsped.org.uk/clinical/docs/DKA ManagementOfDKAinAdultsMarch20101.pdf.

Hasler WL and Chey WD. Nausea and vomiting. *Gastroenterology* 2003; 125: 1860.

Kashani A, Landaverde C, Medici V, and Rossaro L. Fluid retention in cirrhosis: Pathophysiology and management. *Q J Med* 2008; 101: 71–85.

Kidney Disease: Improving Global Outcomes (KDIGO) Acute Kidney Injury Work Group. KDIGO Clinical Practice Guideline for Acute Kidney Injury. *Kidney inter., Suppl.* 2012; 2: 1–138.

Kwan Lai W and Murphy N. Management of acute liver failure. *Contin Educ Anaesth Crit Care Pain* 2004; 4: 40–43.

Latenser BA. Critical care of the burn patient: The first 48 hours. *Crit Care Med* 2009; 37: 2819–26.

Longmore M, Wilkinson I, Baldwin A, and Wallin E. *Oxford Handbook of Clinical Medicine*. 8th Edition. Oxford: Oxford University Press, 2010.

Moller S, Bendtsen F, and Henricksen JH. Pathophysiological basis of pharmacotherapy in the hepatorenal syndrome. *Scand J Gastroenterol* 2005; 40: 491–500.

NICE Guideline 174. *Intravenous fluid therapy in adults in hospital.* https://www.nice.org.uk/guidance/CG174. December 2013.

NICE Guideline 108. *Chronic heart failure in adults: Management.* August 2010. https://www.nice.org.uk/guidance/CG108. August 2010.

NICE Guideline 169. *Prevention, detection and management of acute kidney injury up to the point of renal replacement therapy.* https://www.nice.org.uk/guidance/CG169. August 2013.

Raine, T, Dawson J, Sanders S, and Eccles S. *Oxford Handbook for the Foundation Programme.* 3rd Edition. Oxford: Oxford University Press, 2011.

Ramrakha P and Moore K. *Oxford Handbook of Acute Medicine*. 2nd edition Oxford: Oxford University Press, 2008.

CHAPTER 5

Fluid therapy management in surgical patients

INTRODUCTION

Surgery induces a stress response in human beings; our normal physiology becomes altered, including the fluid and electrolyte equilibrium. Surgical procedures require considerable planning and individualised management before, during and after. Before elective surgery, patients with chronic medical conditions often receive multidisciplinary support to ensure their care is optimised, problems are anticipated and contingency plans are made.

As a junior doctor in a surgical specialty, one is likely to be involved in a pre-assessment clinic, which provides an opportunity to plan for any special requirement the patient may have. For instance, insulin-dependent diabetics may require admission to hospital the day before their procedure, so that a sliding scale can be used to maintain their metabolism while they remain nil-by-mouth (NBM).

During the peri-operative period, the goal is to carefully replace maintenance requirements, insensible losses and extra output like post-operative vomiting. Always consider whether intravenous fluid (IVF) therapy is still required, is the patient's oral intake adequate?

This chapter guides you through the management of fluid balance in patients in the pre- and post-operative periods, addressing special points to consider in certain surgical procedures.

PRE-OPERATIVE FLUID STATUS MANAGEMENT

In some cases, surgical patients are admitted as emergencies, where there is less time for pre-operative assessment and surgery is unavoidable. It is important to focus on resuscitating the patient in these situations (see Chapter 3 for guidance).

Assess the patient's estimated fluid and electrolyte requirements from their history, examination, observations and test results.

History

1. **Planned surgical procedure:** An awareness of the site and extent of surgery will help you predict the patient's likely post-op fluid requirements. Is the procedure likely to be lengthy, increasing the duration of disruption to their usual physiology? For example, a large amount of fluid evaporates from an open abdomen (10–15 mL/kg/hr), so patients having a laparotomy will require extra fluid replacement.

2. **Current fluid status:** Patient's fluid intake and causes of extra fluid losses – do they balance? Ask what the usual fluid intake is like. Do they avoid drinking water? Do they have a fluid restriction (e.g. in renal failure)? Is the daily total intake of fluid adequate? Do they already depend on enteral feeding methods (nasogastric/jejunal)?

   Knowing how often the patient passes urine/self-catheterises/empties their in-dwelling catheter bag/stoma bag will give an estimate of the fluid output.

   Positive (+) fluid balance describes more recorded input than output, whilst negative (–) fluid balance describes more recorded fluid output than input. Determine whether the patient tends towards a positive or negative fluid balance in their routine life before surgery.

REMEMBER

Normal fluid balance
Approximate fluid intake of 70-kg adult:
- 1500-mL liquid
- 750-mL food
- 250-mL product of metabolism
- 2500-mL total

Normal output:
- 1500-mL urine
- 100-mL faeces
- 900-mL insensible loss
- **2500-mL total**

Insensible loss is the unmeasurable volume of pure water lost per day, up to 1200 mL at rest, via the skin and lungs. Tachypnoea, temperature and metabolic rate may increase this level. Loss through sweating is normally negligible but can be greatly increased in, for example, sepsis or hot environments.

3. **Past medical history:** Ask pertinent questions to help guide your pre-operative fluid prescribing; are there any existing conditions that will necessitate cautious prescribing? Do they have a medical condition affecting their body's ability to respond adequately to fluid deficit or excess? Focus on the following:

   a. Cardiovascular – Ischaemic heart disease (IHD) and heart failure (HF) will (in varying degrees) affect the heart's ability to pump blood around the body. Be cautious when prescribing fluid, as decreased cardiac output might result in excess fluid outside the intravascular space.

   b. Renal – Depending on the extent and cause of acute kidney injury (AKI) a patient may require extra fluids, or conversely, require dialysis. Chronic kidney disease (CKD) of varying severity will affect how the body excretes fluids and electrolytes, and hence the quantity and type of fluid required. Patients with end-stage renal failure may not produce urine and may instead require dialysis for offloading of their excess fluid. They may therefore have strict daily fluid input restrictions; volume and type of IVF given peri-operatively should be tailored to this.

   c. Hepatic – Decompensated liver disease may affect sodium and water distribution, so caution should be applied when prescribing fluids, especially sodium-containing fluids like crystalloids.

   d. Gastrointestinal (GI) – Excretion from the GI tract can result in large fluid and electrolyte depletion (especially potassium and sodium), thus high stoma output, diarrhoea and vomiting all require regular electrolyte investigation and aggressive fluid replacement (see Figure 5.1). Compare Table 5.1 with Table 2.1 in Chapter 2. For instance, in a patient with

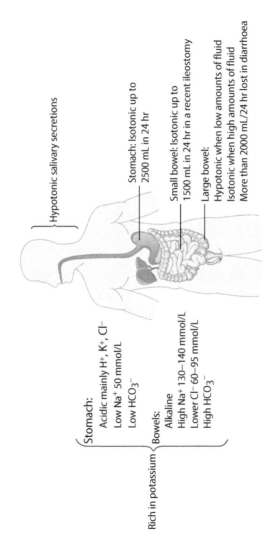

Hypotonic salivary secretions

Stomach: Isotonic up to 2500 mL in 24 hr

Small bowel: Isotonic up to 1500 mL in 24 hr in a recent ileostomy

Large bowel:
Hypotonic when low amounts of fluid
Isotonic when high amounts of fluid
More than 2000 mL/24 hr lost in diarrhoea

Rich in potassium

Stomach:
Acidic mainly H^+, K^+, Cl^-
Low Na^+ 50 mmol/L
Low HCO_3^-

Bowels:
Alkaline
High Na^+ 130–140 mmol/L
Lower Cl^- 60–95 mmol/L
High HCO_3^-

Figure 5.1   Composition of fluids secreted in the GI tract.

Table 5.1   Daily volume and electrolyte composition of gastrointestinal fluids

GI fluid	Volume (mL)	Sodium (mmol/L)	Potassium (mmol/L)	Chloride (mmol/L)	H+ (mmol/L)	HCO₃⁻ (mmol/L)
Gastric	2500	30–80	5–20	100–150	40–60	–
Biliary	500	130	10	100	–	30–50
Pancreatic	1000	130	10	75	–	70–110
Small bowel	5000	130	10	90–130	–	20–40

Source: British National Formulary. https://www.evidence.nhs.uk/formulary/bnf/ current/1-gastro-intestinal-system/16-laxatives/165-bowel-cleansing-preparations/macrogols/klean-prep. Accessed in September 2015.

copious bilious vomiting, around 130 mmol/L of Na^+ is lost in bile daily; this will need replacing with an IVF with a similar sodium content. Hartmann's (131 mmol/L) or 0.9% normal saline (154 mmol/L) can be administered, rather than 5% dextrose, which contains no sodium.

4. **Medication:** Take particular note of medications that affect the function of the heart, kidneys and hormonal control of fluid and electrolyte balance. Some of these medications may need to be omitted or optimised before elective surgery; consult the *British National Formulary* (BNF), a clinical pharmacology text or a senior if you are unsure. The following are common medications in the elderly population and the effects that will influence your management:

a. Angiotensin-converting enzyme (ACE) inhibitors – Renal impairment, first-dose hypotension.

b. Beta-blockers – Can cause decreased cardiac output.

c. Thiazide diuretics – Can cause hypokalaemia, hyponatraemia, oliguria, hyperglycaemia, hypercalcaemia.

d. Loop diuretics – Hypokalaemia, hyponatraemia, hyperglycaemia, hypocalcaemia and dehydration.

e. Potassium-sparing diuretics – Can cause hyperkalaemia, hyponatraemia, water depletion.

f. Calcium-channel blockers – Can cause ankle oedema.

g. Some stimulant laxatives – Can cause dehydration and electrolyte imbalances.

h. Electrolyte supplements – E.g. potassium supplements will increase serum potassium levels.

Examination

Look for clues that suggest decompensation from chronic disease; are there signs of worsening HF for instance, and is there a new-onset arrhythmia?

Weigh the patient to help you establish a baseline estimate of fluid composition; this mostly represents interstitial oedema. During their hospital stay, weighing the patient with the same scales at the same time of day gives an indication of acute hydration status. Maintain a cumulative chart to allow comparison.

Table 5.2 summarises the signs and symptoms associated with altered fluid balance in the pre-operative patient.

In pre-assessment clinics, be sure to pay attention to the blood pressure (BP), heart rate (HR), respiratory rate (RR) and oxygen saturation.

Table 5.2   Signs and symptoms of altered fluid balance in the pre-operative patient

System	Fluid depletion	Fluid overload
Cardiovascular	• Tachycardia • Hypotension • Capillary refill time >2 seconds • Decreased skin turgor • Dry mucous membranes • Postural drop in blood pressure	• Hypertension • Added heart sounds • Raised jugular venous pressure (JVP) • Peripheral/sacral pitting oedema
Respiratory	• Respiratory rate >20 breaths/min	• Oxygen saturation <92% • Respiratory rate >20 breaths/min • Bibasal crackles • Wheeze • Cyanosis
Renal	• Decreased urine output <0.5 mL/kg/hr • Concentrated urine	• Increased urine output >0.5 mL/kg/hr • Clear urine
Gastrointestinal	• Loose stool • High stoma output • Vomiting • Bowel obstruction	

(Continued)

Table 5.2 (*Continued*) Signs and symptoms of altered fluid balance in the pre-operative patient

System	Fluid depletion	Fluid overload
Endocrine	• Blood sugar ≥11 mmol/L • Ketonuria	
Neurological	• Low Glasgow Coma Scale (GCS) <8 • Comatose	• Low GCS <8 • Comatose

If there are abnormal results, their ability to cope with major surgery and fluid and electrolyte balance post-operatively may be affected. Decide if the patient needs a different medication regimen or specialist input before proceeding with surgery.

Investigations

By arranging the appropriate investigations, you play a crucial role in optimising the patient for surgery and recovery; for instance, a simple blood test could reveal that the patient's condition has led to hypokalaemia, easily corrected with oral supplementation in the days before surgery.

1. **Blood tests:** Especially important are up-to-date measurements and review of the patient's urea, electrolytes, liver function tests (LFTs) and haemoglobin (Hb). For instance, a woman with heavy periods may become severely anaemic while awaiting a hysterectomy; she may need a pre-operative red blood cell transfusion (see Chapter 6).

   Urea and creatinine are often assessed together, to help determine current renal function. These need to be closely monitored if a patient has known chronic renal impairment; persistently abnormal levels may necessitate dialysis in the peri-operative period.

   Normal urea 2.5–8.0 mmol/L.

   Normal creatinine 64–104 μmol/L (males) and 49–90 μmol/L (females).

   a. Raised urea can be caused by sepsis and GI bleeding (high-protein load).

   b. Raised urea disproportionate to, or without raised creatinine can be caused by hypovolaemia leading to pre-renal failure. Rises in both can be caused by chronic kidney failure.

   c. Estimated glomerular filtration rate (eGFR) may also be useful.

2. **Electrocardiogram:** Essential for assessment of any current cardiac ischaemia or rhythm abnormality: Fluid therapy will depend on the extent and cause of the problem. Where possible look at previous electrocardiograms (ECGs) and compare for any signs of atrial fibrillation, myocardial infarction or dysrhythmias.

3. **Imaging:** Useful to help determine if there is abnormal fluid distribution, such as chest x-ray (CXR) findings in the case of pulmonary oedema. Furthermore, imaging allows investigation into the clinical cause of abnormal fluid distribution, such as a cardiac or renal abnormality.

   a. Radiographs – CXR for any signs of fluid overload
   b. Echocardiogram – Left ventricular ejection fraction (LVEF), ventricular enlargement, dysfunctional pumping
   c. Ultrasound scan – Renal hydronephrosis, small kidneys, and renal cysts/carcinoma
   d. Computed tomography (CT) – CT of the abdomen for bowel obstruction and perforation and CT of the chest for chronic pleural effusions and empyema

Management

In elective surgery, the *Enhanced Recovery Programme* aims to minimise the body's stress response to anaesthesia and surgery, reducing post-operative recovery time. This method is now widely used across many surgical specialties and central to its ethos is the management of fluid balance and fasting times, to help avoid dehydration and malnutrition.

Treat the underlying cause

In a surgical specialty, the appropriate management choice may vary according to the patient's clinical status, i.e. patients who are initially managed conservatively may show worsening of their symptoms and therefore need urgent surgical management instead. In bowel obstruction for instance, nasogastric (NG) tube drainage or decompression at sigmoidoscopy may be required to relieve fluid and electrolyte loss via vomiting.

Treat the current fluid status

As part of the *Enhanced Recovery Programme*, surgical patients are often given one or two clear, carbohydrate-rich drinks (Preload®) before midnight and another drink 2–3 hours before surgery to help ease symptoms of fasting and hunger. They are also thought to contribute to a quicker return to normal bowel function and minimise loss of body mass via anaerobic metabolism. Diabetic patients should be given these drinks along with their usual medications.

A fluid balance chart should be maintained by nursing staff, especially in unwell patients, in whom you should also consider placing a urinary catheter. If recorded accurately, these measures will be invaluable in helping you, the junior doctor, to detect when there is an imbalance in a patient's fluid input and output. Does the rate of the infusion need to be altered? Perhaps sips of clear fluids are adequate now?

Daily replacement of maintenance fluid and electrolytes whilst a patient is fasting does not usually exceed 3 L and this should be reduced to 2–2.5 L in those who are frail, elderly, malnourished or have existing renal or cardiac impairment. Calculations for obese patients (BMI >40 kg/m^2) should be based on their ideal and not actual body weight.

REMEMBER

When a patient is NBM, the following symptoms and signs may develop:

- Dehydration
- Nausea and vomiting
- Electrolyte imbalance
- Hypoglycaemia
- Malnutrition

Aim to match their background maintenance requirements: 25–30 mL/kg/day of water, up to 40 mL/kg/day in healthy young adults **and** approximately 1 mmol/kg/day of potassium, sodium and chloride.

Don't ever forget the glucose! Approximately 50–100 g/day is required to limit starvation ketosis.

Alternating 1-L Hartmann's and 5% dextrose infusions over the fasted period in a healthy person is usually sufficient, but adjust the rate according to individual need. Previous teaching of '1 salty, 2 sweet' is now outdated.

Isotonic IVFs like 0.9% normal saline provide adequate water and electrolytes, but no glucose. In cases where prolonged pre-operative starvation occurs, the body will need more balanced solutions to avoid hyperchloraemic acidosis and hypoglycaemia. Maintenance requirements can be met by providing water, sodium and potassium, as is found in Hartmann's solution or Plasmalyte. The brain, renal medulla and red cells can get energy from stored sugar or protein from muscle breakdown, but these are unsustainable in prolonged starvation. Hypotonic solutions like 5% dextrose can be used intermittently to provide glucose (but not electrolytes) in prolonged starvation.

Excessive losses from gastric aspiration or vomiting should be treated pre-operatively with a balanced crystalloid solution that contains potassium, such as Hartmann's solution, Ringer's solution or Plasmalyte. Losses from diarrhoea/ileostomy/small bowel fistula/ileus/obstruction should be replaced volume-for-volume with Hartmann's or Ringer's lactate type of solutions.

Patients can take the following before being anaesthetised (check with a senior or the anaesthetist on your surgical list if unsure. Local guidelines may provide similar information):

Adult: Water up to 2 hours before anaesthesia (encourage moistened mouth swabs). Food up to 6 hours before.

Child: Water and clear fluids up to 2 hours before anaesthesia. Breast milk up to 4 hours before. Formula/cow's milk or solids up to 6 hours before.

Review the implemented treatment

Although the pre-operative patient is now in the ward, awaiting surgery, it is not good practice to simply prescribe a litre of a generic infusion and leave them to it! You must monitor them closely for warning signs of fluid overload, dehydration, altered consciousness or other adverse outcome.

Sick surgical inpatients must have regular blood tests; review the urea, creatinine, electrolyte and Hb levels on a flowchart if possible. Cumulative analysis helps you pick up abnormal trends much more quickly. Encourage the nursing staff to use the hospital's *Early warning chart* to record all observations and alert you if the system triggers.

For example, if a patient's BP suddenly drops to 80/50 mmHg and remains low despite the nurse repositioning them, do not hesitate to switch the infusing crystalloid for a 500- or 250-mL challenge of an intravascular volume-expanding colloid like *Volplex*. Stay with the patient until you notice sustained improvement in the observations and urine output, think about possible causes of the sudden change and address them. Causes of such sudden changes could include sepsis or hypovolaemia.

Special considerations

Some operations require special preparation for the patient; for instance, low fibre and then bowel preparations are used to empty the bowels before a colonoscopy or colonic surgery. Commonly administered bowel preparations include oral sodium phosphate and *Klean-Prep*. These are designed to minimise dehydration but have the additional effect of inducing GI electrolyte losses and fluid imbalance. The high sodium and phosphate content makes these solutions hyperosmolar; they cause water to be retained in the intestinal lumen, leading to peristalsis and colonic emptying. *Klean-Prep* contains large macrogol molecules which remain in the bowel lumen, exerting an osmotic effect that keeps water within the lumen, softening stool and making it easier to pass. To achieve this, bowel preparation sachets are mixed with large volumes of water, up to 4 L over split doses. In the elderly, frail or in those with renal or HF, this volume is reduced to around 2 L in total, to avoid interstitial oedema.

Bowel preparations have the added side effect of inducing dehydration, hyponatraemia and hypokalaemia. Check the patient's electrolyte levels and fluid balance after bowel preparation is used; correct with titrated volumes of intravenous 0.9% normal saline or balanced crystalloid (Hartmann's or Plasmalyte) as necessary.

In *chronic renal failure*, there is associated electrolyte imbalance and reduced diuresis, hence the importance of estimating the patient's usual urine output and checking the electrolytes pre-operatively. Aim to balance the fluids to at least match the usual urine output and avoid blind addition of potassium, as hyperkalaemia can develop. In a healthy person, at least 400 mL of daily urine clearance is required to maintain normal function; in a person with renal failure, much less urine is produced. Avoid using arteriovenous (AV) fistulas, cephalic and subclavian veins to administer fluids or take blood samples as these need to be protected for dialysis.

KLEAN-PREP

Each sachet of Klean-Prep contains the following active ingredients:

Macrogol 3350	59.000 g
Anhydrous sodium sulphate	5.685 g
Sodium bicarbonate	1.685 g
Sodium chloride	1.465 g
Potassium chloride	0.7425 g

The content of electrolyte ions per sachet when made up to 1 L with water is as follows:

Sodium	125 mmol/L
Sulphate	40 mmol/L
Chloride	35 mmol/L
Bicarbonate	20 mmol/L
Potassium	10 mmol/L

Source: British National Formulary. https://www.evidence.nhs.uk/formulary/bnf/current/1-gastro-intestinal-system/16-laxatives/165-bowel-cleaning-preparations/macrogols/klean-prep. Accessed September 2015. With permission.

INTRA-OPERATIVE FLUID BALANCE

During surgery higher volumes of fluid are lost as a result of fluid compartment shift in response to surgical trauma. Extracellular fluid from the intravascular space moves to the interstitial space producing oedema of the bowel wall and mesentery, along with oedema of subcutaneous tissue and muscle. Evaporative loss is also increased, especially during open abdominal surgery. Estimates for intra-operative fluid replacement are as follows:

- 2–5 mL/kg/hr for superficial or peripheral surgeries
- 5–10 mL/kg/hr for open abdominal or thoracic surgeries
- 10–15 mL/kg/hr for major open abdominal surgery

During surgery, further fluid loss comes from loss of blood, mechanical ventilation (respiratory tract) and evaporation from skin in those who are pyrexial. An added aid to assessment of intra-operative fluid status is the oesophageal Doppler, now widely used to achieve 'goal-directed' fluid therapy. This term relates to using restrictive amounts of IVF and advanced haemodynamic monitoring to maintain euvolaemia rather than hypervolaemia as previously taught. There is some evidence that goal-directed fluid therapy helps to maintain tissue perfusion and reduce complication rates and post-operative hospital stay (see GIFTASUP in the 'Further reading' section at the end of this chapter). Also lookout for outcomes of the ongoing RELIEF trial (large multi-centre analysis of restrictive versus liberal fluid therapy in major abdominal surgery).

As a junior doctor looking after the post-surgical patient, it is useful to review the anaesthetic chart to determine how the patient's fluid balance was managed intra-operatively. For instance, intra-operatively, a patient with obstructive jaundice should have had judicious fluid replacement and diuretics to help prevent AKI secondary to hepatorenal syndrome. This will have an influence on how you manage the patient's fluid balance immediately after surgery.

POST-OPERATIVE FLUID STATUS MANAGEMENT

Patients are at risk of complications associated with their operation directly (haemorrhage) or indirectly (infection, thrombosis), early signs of which can be detected by the vigilant junior doctor. The first 24 hours post-surgery are crucial, as oral intake is limited and the body has higher requirements to help it re-adjust.

Antidiuretic hormone (ADH) and renin–angiotensin–aldosterone system products are released after surgery, leading to water retention. Stress hormones including cortisol, adrenaline and glucagon as well as inflammatory mediators are released, increasing vascular permeability and interstitial fluid retention. Physiological organ functions are impaired, including renal clearance of excess electrolytes. In addition, potassium is released by damaged tissues; it accumulates if renal perfusion and therefore urine output is impaired, leading to the risk of arrhythmias. Potassium supplementation is often not required in the first 24 hours after surgery for this reason.

Post-operatively, if surgery was straightforward, patients should only need IVF therapy for a short period until they are able to resume a normal diet (encouraged within 24 hours if on an *Enhanced Recovery Programme*). Other reasons for giving post-operative IVF include to manage hypovolaemia, avoid renal failure, and to minimise hypotension secondary to regional anaesthesia and analgesia. In those who require IVF for maintenance in the immediate post-operative period, choose a solution that has lower sodium and at as low a volume as possible. This is because the body is already holding on to sodium and water as a physiological response to the stress of surgery. Consider administering 4% dextrose/0.18% normal saline for this reason.

In the situation where the patient is unlikely to resume a normal diet within 5–7 days, e.g. bowel rest in colostomy formation, nutritional support will be required. This could be via the enteral route (NG, nasojejunal, percutaneous endoscopic gastrostomy tubes) or central/peripheral total parenteral nutrition.

History

Ask about: Ability to eat and drink. Are they only tolerating sips of water or more?

- Vomiting: Frequency and amount. NG drain output.
- Urinary output: Frequency, colour and amount.
- Bowel movements: Flatus, diarrhoea, stoma output if relevant.
- Wound drain output: Volume and character.

Loss of water through the GI tract is increased in diarrhoea and when there is an ileostomy, as there is no colonic water reabsorption. A basic knowledge of the procedure the patient has had is essential in helping you anticipate the likely post-operative course/recovery of the patient.

1. **Current fluid status:** Positive (+) fluid balance describes more recorded input than output, whilst negative (-) fluid balance describes more recorded fluid output than input.

2. **Past medical history:** If the patient is conscious, ask about any existing conditions that will necessitate cautious prescribing? Do they have a medical condition which will affect their body's ability to respond adequately to fluid deficit or excess? Review the medical notes if you do not already know the patient, looking for cardiovascular, renal and GI conditions in particular (review the History section under the 'Pre-Operative Fluid Status Management' section of this chapter).

3. **Medication:** In the immediate post-operative period, patients may not be alert/stable enough to take their usual medications and they are exposed to new drugs such as analgesics, diuretics and anti-emetics. Take particular note of medications that

affect the function of the heart, kidneys and hormonal control of fluid and electrolyte balance. For example, do not blindly restart diuretics or nonsteroidal anti-inflammatory (NSAIDs) without an examination and check of the renal function, as this may lead to AKI.

Examination

Look for clues that suggest that the patient is not coping with the insult of anaesthesia and surgery, or is developing a complication. Are they able to maintain perfusion? Do they have difficulty breathing? Is there a new onset of confusion?

If possible, weigh the patient daily for added information on fluid balance, and maintain a cumulative chart to allow comparison, especially in cardiac patients. Check for signs of fluid overload. Is there pitting oedema? Crepitations/crackles on lung auscultation?

As well as conducting a systematic examination as for the pre-operative patient, look for clues about altered fluid balance in the post-operative patient:

- Skin colour and turgor. Does the patient appear pale/mottled? Do the peripheries feel warm or cold?
- Inspect the urinary catheter. Does urine appear concentrated/diluted? Is there bloodstaining or frank haematuria? What is the volume of urine within the bag? How often has it been emptied?
- Inspect the wound drain(s) if present. Haemoserous fluid or frank blood? Is the fluid leaking out of the drain insertion site? What is the total volume drained since insertion?
- Inspect and palpate the surgical site looking for signs of ongoing bleeding: tense, tender abdomen, widespread bruising across the lower back, swollen joints.
- Inspect the NG tube/stoma bag if present; what are the contents like? Volume drained?

Investigations

Most patients do not need investigations during their hospital stay after an operation; however, if there is deviation from the expected recovery course (as suggested by the history and examination), appropriate investigations such as radiographs, ultrasound, CT, ECG and echocardiogram become useful.

Blood tests: Especially important are an up-to-date measurement of the patient's Hb, urea, electrolyte and LFT levels. Surgery alters the body's biochemical and hormonal balance; fluids and electrolytes shift, and stroke volume, microvascular blood flow and tissue oxygen delivery is altered.

- Check the full blood count (FBC) within 12–24 hours if dealing with a major surgical procedure such as a gastrectomy, colectomy or hysterectomy. If the patient shows signs of being unwell, serial FBC checks 6 hours apart are useful to determine whether further intervention such as transfusion (replace lost blood) or return to theatre (stem ongoing bleeding) are required. Hemocue can be used as a simple bedside test to determine if there has been a drop in Hb.

Management

Post-operatively, most patients are in a fluid-depleted state, owing to pre-operative starvation, vomiting, and intra-operative blood and insensible fluid loss. The focus of management is to replace this deficit within the first 24 hours (may require up to 4–5 L) and then return to maintenance levels (2–3 L/day) if they still require IVF. Aim to avoid fluid overload by also checking that their normal body weight is maintained and overall fluid balance is near zero. In a more monitored setting, lactate, mean arterial pressure (MAP) and urine output are used as measures of adequate fluid repletion and maintenance; aim for MAP ≥65 mmHg, urine output ≥0.5 mL/kg/hr and if available, central venous oxygen saturation of 70%.

A fluid balance chart should be maintained by nursing staff, especially in unwell patients, who should also have a urinary catheter. If recorded accurately, these measures will be invaluable in helping you, the junior doctor, to detect when there is an imbalance in a patient's fluid input and output. Does the rate of the infusion need to be altered? Perhaps sips of clear fluids are adequate now? Watch out for signs of re-feeding syndrome when the patient starts to take solid food after a prolonged period of reliance on IVF (see Case 1 in Chapter 4).

Isotonic IVF like 0.9% normal saline risks hypernatraemia/hyperchloraemia. Hyperchloraemia has the effect of reduced splanchnic and renal blood flow, as well as exacerbation of the inflammatory response in sepsis. Hartmann's provides adequate water and electrolytes and acts as an alkaline buffer in acidosis (sepsis, hypovolaemia). However, as hypovolaemia is common post-operatively, colloids like *Volpex* may be required to maintain intravascular volume and therefore cardiac stroke volume and tissue perfusion to also aid healing.

REMEMBER

When a patient is NBM, the following symptoms and signs may develop:

- Dehydration
- Nausea and vomiting
- Electrolyte imbalance
- Hypoglycaemia
- Malnutrition

Aim to replace the depleted fluid volume and electrolytes at a rate of around 1.5 mL/kg/hr, adjusted according to clinical status.

Then aim to match their background maintenance requirements:

25–30 mL/kg/day of water in the elderly, up to 40 mL/kg/day in healthy young adults and approximately 1 mmol/kg/day of potassium, sodium and chloride.

Don't ever forget the glucose! Approximately 50–100 g/day is required to limit starvation ketosis.

Alternating 1-L Hartmann's and 5% dextrose infusions over the post-operative NBM period in a healthy person is usually sufficient, but adjust the rate according to individual need. Consider administering 4% dextrose/0.18% normal saline in the immediate post-operative period.

Peri-operative blood loss of large volumes, i.e. greater than 500 mL, may need to be replaced with transfusion of red blood cells/fresh frozen plasma, etc. if the patient remains symptomatic despite volume replacement with colloids or balanced crystalloids. The patient should be counselled appropriately and steps taken to ensure safe transfusion.

The brain, renal medulla and red cells can get energy from stored sugar or protein from muscle breakdown, but these are unsustainable. Hypotonic solutions like 5% dextrose provide sugar but not electrolytes; they drive water into the intracellular space, increasing the risk of iatrogenic hyponatraemia and peripheral oedema if used for prolonged periods. A solution of 4% dextrose/0.18% normal saline is a more appropriate post-operative fluid as this corrects sodium and water depletion. Most water moves down its osmotic gradient into the intracellular space, glucose also moves into the cell and the sodium mainly remains in the extracellular space.

Review the implemented treatment

You must monitor the patient closely for warning signs of fluid overload, dehydration, altered consciousness or other adverse outcome.

Post-operative inpatients whose recovery is not straightforward must have regular blood tests; review the urea, creatinine, electrolyte and Hb levels on a flowchart if possible. Cumulative analysis helps you pick up abnormal trends much more quickly. Encourage the nursing staff to use the hospital's *Early warning chart* to record all observations and alert you if the system triggers. Cumulative analysis of blood results and fluid balance charts helps you adjust your choice of IVF and flow rate, and eventually stop therapy altogether.

As mentioned previously, if a patient's BP suddenly drops to 80/50 mmHg and remains low despite the nurse repositioning them, do not hesitate to switch the infusing crystalloid for a 500- or 250-mL challenge of an intravascular volume-expanding colloid like *Volplex*. Stay with the patient until you notice sustained improvement in their observations, think about possible causes of the sudden change and address them. Perhaps there is ongoing intra-abdominal bleeding. Look for other signs, re-examine the patient and call for additional support from team members early on.

If a blood transfusion was required, have you checked an FBC and clotting profile 6 hours or more after completion? Do you need the support of a specialist nurse/dietician? Is the patient now stable enough to return to a normal diet and be discharged home?

Serial blood gases may display a rising lactate level, a subtle sign of worsening hypoperfusion.

Special considerations

Paralytic ileus is a post-operative problem which usually resolves within 48 hours. Manipulation of the bowel, sympathetic system action and potassium depletion contribute to its development. It features abdominal distension, vomiting, constipation and absence of intestinal movements. Loss of large volumes of fluid, electrolytes (especially potassium) and protein into the gut lumen occurs (third-space losses), which should be carefully replaced. If the patient remains NBM, they may require an NG tube draining gastric fluids and a urinary catheter. IVF (0.9% normal saline with 20–40-mmol potassium chloride or Hartmann's solution), gut motility agents (e.g. metoclopramide) and analgesia are the mainstay of treatment (drip and suck). Be sure to monitor the fluid balance and daily serum electrolyte levels, adjusting the volume and type of IVF given accordingly.

Ascitic drainage carries a risk of hypovolaemia, hypoalbuminaemia and electrolyte disturbances ($\downarrow K^+$, $\downarrow Na^+$). Minimise these risks and detect by draining no more than 500–1000 mL/hr, maintaining a strict input/output fluid balance chart and checking observations at least every 4 hours. Aim to correct signs of hypovolaemia quickly, with a colloid (malignant ascites) or human albumin solution (from haematology, in portal-hypertensive ascites).

Irrigating solutions are used in endoscopic operations like transurethral resection of the prostate/bladder tumours, transcervical resection of the endometrium, cystoscopy and arthroscopy. The aim is to help distend the operative field and wash away debris. Solutions used alongside monopolar electrocautery contain one or two solutes; glycine (amino acid), mannitol (glucose isomer) and sorbitol (fructose and sucrose). Solutions used alongside bipolar electrocautery or in the absence of electricity contain electrolytes; sterile water or normal saline.

There is a risk of absorption of irrigating fluid into the vascular system and then body tissues, leading to a collection of symptoms known as 'transurethral syndrome' – hyponatraemia, hyperkalaemia, cerebral oedema, renal failure, and/or bradycardia and hypotension progressing to pulmonary oedema. Although rare, this occurs more with use of glycine, in transurethral resection of the prostate (TURP) and transcervical resection of the endometrium (TCRE), up to 3-L absorption in some reported cases. Treatment is supportive and involves fluid restriction, diuretics and observation. Correct the hyponatraemia (<120 mmol/L) slowly with hypertonic saline (7.5%) at a rate of 1 mmol/L/hr to achieve a serum sodium level of 130 mmol/L.

Ileostomies are used to manage conditions such as large bowel obstruction, malignancy or inflammatory bowel disease. As previously mentioned, the small bowel secretes a high volume of fluid (approximately 5000 mL) rich in sodium, chloride, potassium and enzymes in the healthy state. In those with ileostomies, this may be more pronounced, especially when first sited. The absorption of certain vitamins and minerals can also be diminished. Maintain a strict fluid input–output chart whilst the patient is in hospital and check electrolyte levels and renal function daily. If the patient is constantly in negative fluid balance, they will require large volumes of oral or IVF replacement, and in some cases, anti-motility agents and soluble fibre supplements to bulk up the ileostomy output. Select an IVF such as Hartmann's or Plasmalyte, which both have adequate sodium and potassium levels. Continue to monitor response to fluids and titrate volume and selection of fluid according to this.

CONCLUSION

Surgery produces a physiological stress response in the human body. As a junior doctor, you can help the patient prepare for this disruption to normal function and reduce the risk of morbidity and mortality perioperatively. Starting at admission or in the pre-assessment clinic, use your history-taking and examination skills to determine if your patient has pre-existing risk factors such as cardiopulmonary disease, renal failure or coagulation disorders. Use the *Enhanced Recovery Programme* protocol to guide your management. Aim to match the body's maintenance fluid requirements in the pre-operative NBM period (25–30 mL/kg/day of water, up to 40 mL/kg/day in healthy young adults and approximately 1 mmol/kg/day of potassium, sodium and chloride).

Intra-operatively, match maintenance requirements and aim to replace lost fluid volume from the surgical procedure. The patient may be hypovolaemic and hypotensive after surgery, requiring larger volumes of IVF. 4% dextrose/0.18% normal saline is a reasonable choice in the immediate post-operative period; switch to balanced crystalloids or colloids depending on the patient's response. Once the patient tolerates sips of water, stop IVF therapy. Familiarise yourself with the common surgical procedures conducted in your particular specialty, so that you can understand why certain procedures may need slightly different fluid therapy regimes.

CASE 5.1 – PANCREATITIS

A 72-year-old man is referred to the surgical assessment ward with a 2-day history of worsening 'pain at the breastbone'. This did not resolve with simple painkillers and he has now started vomiting, with an associated fever. He states that he had a procedure to remove gallstones recently; you check his discharge letter and discover that this was an endoscopic retrograde cholangiopancreatography (ERCP) done 2 weeks previously. Otherwise, he has no chronic medical conditions nor does he take any regular medications.

Airway: Patent. He is able to complete full sentences, but he winces during conversation.

Breathing: He prefers to sit upright, with his arms braced against the examination couch. No abnormal breath sounds auscultated. RR 26 breaths/min. Oxygen saturation 94% on air.

Circulation: Clammy, cool peripheries, capillary refill time (CRT) 4 seconds. HR 100 bpm. BP 110/70. Some difficulty establishing a patent cannula, but a 16G cannula is eventually sited and blood taken for arterial blood gas (ABG) and FBC, urea and electrolytes (U+Es), LFTs, amylase, clotting profile and group and save sampling.

Disability: Glasgow Coma Scale (GCS) score 15/15. Capillary blood glucose level is 11.5 mmol/L. Urinalysis shows a trace of glucose and ketones.

Exposure: On inspection there is mild jaundice of the sclera, and mild abdominal distension. The abdomen is generally tender, but more so in the right upper quadrant. Digital rectal exam revealed no abnormalities.

What is the main abnormality and what is the most likely underlying diagnosis?

This patient presents with a variety of problems: abdominal pain following ERCP, vomiting, jaundice, hyperglycaemia, fever and signs of developing shock. Overall, the fact that his illness has developed soon after ERCP suggests acute pancreatitis. Diagnostic criteria for acute pancreatitis include the following:

- Sudden onset of persistent, severe epigastric or generalised abdominal pain radiating to the back.
- Elevation of serum lipase or amylase to more than three times the upper limit of normal.

CASE 5.1 (continued)

- Features of pancreatic/peritoneal inflammation on imaging such as transabdominal ultrasound, CT or MRI. Imaging is only recommended if there is diagnostic uncertainty.

What are your priorities in treating this patient?
As this patient is already starting to show signs of severe pancreatitis and shock, he should be admitted to an acute surgical bed with regular checks of his BP, HR, RR, temperature and oxygen saturation. Resuscitation should include IVF therapy and supplemental oxygen to maintain his oxygen saturation at 94%–98%.

Hallmarks

- Severe acute abdominal pain, sometimes localised to the epigastrium.
- Markedly raised amylase or lipase or both, secondary to leakage from the inflamed pancreas into the systemic circulation.
- More commonly caused by gallstones or alcohol.
- Grey Turner's sign occurs late and rarely in the disease process; bruised appearance of the loins due to retroperitoneal tracking of bloodstained pancreatic juice.
- Severe pancreatitis features marked hypovolaemic shock; toxins from the inflamed pancreas and the body's inflammatory response make capillary walls leakier; water and sodium leak out of the intravascular space and into surrounding tissues. Tissue hypoperfusion and end-organ failure also feature.

Investigations

- ABG/venous blood gases (VBGs) provide information on acid–base status, tissue perfusion and electrolyte imbalance.
- Blood tests including LFTs, U+Es, amylase, FBC.
- ECG may show abnormalities secondary to electrolyte imbalance.
- Gallstones may cause obstruction of the ampulla of the pancreas or oedema of the pancreatic head; investigate/manage with ERCP or magnetic resonance cholangiopancreatography (MRCP) perhaps after the acute phase has settled.

Management

Supportive treatment includes analgesia, antibiotics, resting the pancreas by being NBM, and IVF replacement. To determine the severity of pancreatitis and therefore the management, use a scoring system such as Glasgow criteria or Acute Physiology and Chronic Health Evaluation II (APACHE II) score. A patient with a high score has a more severe form of pancreatitis, with a higher risk of mortality, so they should be managed in an intensive care setting.

Hypovolaemia in pancreatitis can progress quickly to shock and cardiovascular collapse; fluid replacement, particularly within the first 24 hours has been shown to reduce mortality. A balanced crystalloid is ideal in the initial stages, but adjust the volume and choice of fluid in accordance with the patient's response to treatment. Maintain MAP at 65–85 mmHg, urine output >0.5 mL/kg/hr. Monitor the observations and blood glucose every hour; hyperglycaemia may need treatment if persistent. U+Es should be checked at least once a day to guide treatment.

CASE 5.2 – BOWEL OBSTRUCTION

Meg is a 42-year-old nulliparous woman currently undergoing investigations for abdominal bloating. She has had a negative urine pregnancy test, her general practitioner (GP) has asked her to keep a food diary and she is awaiting a transabdominal ultrasound. She presents to the urgent care centre with a history of increasing abdominal pain and bloating, as well as a new onset of vomiting. Her observations are within normal limits; serum blood test results of note are as follows:

Hb 112 g/L	Na$^+$ 130 mmol/L	LFTs are within normal limits
WCC 11 × 10^9	K$^+$ 4 mmol/L	
Neutrophils 4 × 10^9	Creatinine 65 μmol/L	
CRP 50	Urea 10 mmol/L	

On assessment, she is noted to have dry mucous membranes, reduced skin turgor and a tense, distended and generally tender abdomen. She vomits around 400 mL of bilious fluid during the consultation and she does not recall when she last passed urine.

What is the main abnormality and what is the most likely underlying diagnosis?

Gradual development of abdominal distension has developed into acute abdominal pain and vomiting. Meg is also showing signs of dehydration. An AXR in A&E is likely to confirm small bowel obstruction. Further investigations may be required to determine the exact cause of obstruction.

CASE 5.2 (continued)

What are your priorities in treating this patient?

As Meg is in acute pain and showing signs of dehydration, she will need resuscitation with IVF and analgesia. This warrants hospital admission and assessment by a member of the surgical on-call team. Once resuscitated, she will need further assessment to help determine whether surgical intervention is required or not; this may include decompression of dilated bowel, reducing intussusception or resecting ischaemic bowel.

Hallmarks

- Vomiting, cramping/paroxysmal abdominal pain, inability to pass stool or flatus
- Signs of dehydration including hypotension, tachycardia, reduced urine output
- Tinkling or reduced bowel sounds in mechanical obstruction

Investigations

- Blood tests have already been done. A lactate level would be a useful indicator of tissue perfusion and likelihood of infection.
- AXR/erect CXR may show dilated bowel loops, intra-abdominal mass, air under the diaphragm suggestive of bowel perforation.
- More detailed imaging via CT may be required to identify the underlying cause of obstruction.

Management

In small bowel obstruction, there is dilatation of bowel loops proximal to the point of obstruction and collapse of bowel distal to this point. Fluid accumulates within the bowel lumen, distending it. The bowel walls become oedematous, and their absorptive function is diminished. Vomiting leads to loss of sodium, chloride, potassium and hydrogen ions from the body, resulting in hypovolaemia and signs of hypotension.

An NG tube helps to drain and decompress the build-up of fluid; however, it is not always tolerated by conscious patients. The patient most often remains NBM to avoid aggravating the obstruction.

Replacement IVF therapy aims to replace lost intravascular fluid volume and electrolytes especially potassium. Like-for-like volume replacement with some additional volume to account for insensible losses is advised, especially as patients can lose a significant amount of fluid through vomiting. Hartmann's solution,

Ringer's lactate or 0.9% normal saline with added potassium chloride are advised. Titrate the volume given to the patient's responses: are BP, HR and urine output normalising? Are the serum potassium and sodium levels within normal limits?

Some patients improve with conservative management (drip and suck), gradually the vomiting and abdominal pain eases and they are able to tolerate oral intake again. Others may deteriorate into hypovolaemic shock and cardiac arrest, especially if there is sudden bowel perforation or ischaemia. Resuscitation and then surgical intervention may be required.

Further reading

British National Formulary. https://www.evidence.nhs.uk/formulary/bnf/current/ 9-nutrition-and-blood/92-fluids-and-electrolytes. Accessed in September 2015.

British National Formulary. https://www.evidence.nhs.uk/formulary/bnf/current/1-gastro-intestinal-system/16-laxatives/165-bowel-cleansing-preparations/macrogols/klean-prep. Accessed in September 2015.

Catherine Liddle. https://www.nursingtimes.net/roles/nurse-educators/nil-by-mouth-best-practice-and-patient-education/5072184.article.

Desborough JP. The stress response to surgery. *Br J Anaesth* 2000; 85: 109–117.

Ellis HE, Christopher JEW and Roy C. *Lecture Notes: General Surgery*, 11th Edition. Oxford, UK: John Wiley (original), 2006.

Goldberg A and Stansby G. *Surgical Talk: Revision in Surgery*, 2nd Edition. London: Imperial College Press, 2005.

Gupta R, Gan TJ, Mythen MG, et al. The World Congress on Enhanced Recovery 2015 conference summary. *Anesth Analg* 2016; 122(3): 911–913. doi:10.1213/ANE.0000000000001149.

Hahn RG. *Clinical Fluid Therapy in the Perioperative Setting*, 1st Edition. Cambridge: Cambridge University Press, 2011.

Heher EC, Thier SO, Rennke H, Humphreys BD. Adverse renal and metabolic effects associated with oral sodium phosphate bowel preparation. *Clin J Am Soc Nephrol* 2008; 3(5): 1494–1503.

KLEAN-PREP. https://www.medicines.org.uk/emc/medicine/1243.

Leeds University Hospitals. http://www.pathology.leedsth.nhs.uk/pathology/Portals/0/Policies/ClinBiochem/BP-2011-08.pdf.

Minto G and Mythen MG. Peri-operative fluid management: Science, art or random chaos? *Br J Anaesth* 2015; 114(5): 717–721. doi:10.1093/bja/aev067.

NICE Guildeline. *Intravenous fluid therapy in adults in hospital.* 174. December 2013.

Park GR and Roe PG. *Fluid Balance and Volume Resuscitation for Beginners.* Greenwich Medical Media, 2000.

Pestana CP. *Fluids and Electrolytes in the Surgical Patient*, 5th Edition. Lippincott Williams & Wilkins, 2000.

Powell-Tuck J, Gosling P, Lobo DN, et al. British Consensus Guidelines on Intravenous Fluid Therapy for Adult Surgical Patients, March 2011. http://www.bapen.org.uk/pdfs/bapen_pubs/giftasup.pdf.

The Royal College of Surgeons. *The Higher Risk General Surgical Patient: Towards Improved Care for a Forgotten Group.* London: RCSENG – Professional Standards and Regulation, 2011.

Scott MJ and Fawcett WJ. Oral carbohydrate preload drink for major surgery – the first steps from famine to feast. *Anaesthesia* 2014; 69(12): 1308–1313.

CHAPTER 6

Blood products and transfusion

INTRODUCTION

As a junior doctor, you are expected to recognise clinical indicators for transfusion of blood components, counsel the patient and gain their consent for this. You will also prescribe, organise and sometimes oversee the administration of blood.

When assessing a patient who is being considered for transfusion, aim to determine what the cause of bleeding is. Is it chronic or acute? Is there an intrinsic problem with the production of cells or clotting factors? Is there over-coagulation requiring reversal? Ensure that you are taking steps to prevent further blood loss and/or anaemia, and resuscitate the patient if signs of shock are present. Once you have assessed the patient for signs and symptoms of anaemia, if you remain unsure about whether a transfusion is necessary, discuss with a senior member of your team or a haematologist. Always consider whether alternatives to extrinsic blood products are more suitable. In some cases, such as Jehovah's Witnesses and oncology patients, the risks of transfusion can outweigh the benefits. Alternatives include colloid fluid, iron replacement and autologous transfusion/cell saver techniques.

After you have determined that a patient would benefit from a transfusion, you must discuss the indication, process, risks and intended outcome with them if they are conscious. This should include sharing written information (local hospital or national leaflet) and documenting verbal consent to proceed. If the patient is unconscious or if major trauma has occurred, you may not be able to converse with the patient, but act in their best interests and transfuse if necessary to save their life.

Transfused blood components contribute to the circulating fluid volume and can lead to transfusion-associated circulatory overload. It is therefore essential to consider the patient's individual attributes; weight, elderly age and concomitant medical problems such as heart failure (HF) and renal impairment. Consider whether a slower rate of administration is required, is a diuretic required after transfusion, and if so, at which stage? Check for signs of fluid overload during transfusion.

This chapter aims to revise the clinical assessment of acute anaemia, available blood products and their indications/cautions, common transfusion regimes, as well as special cases to consider.

ASSESSMENT

Symptoms of anaemia are commonly non-specific and in the case of chronic anaemia, can be absent. With a gradual decline in haemoglobin (Hb), the body is able to compensate and increase the oxygen-carrying capacity of blood; however, with acute blood loss patients tend to decompensate more quickly, developing hypovolaemia and symptoms such as dizziness, fatigue, irritability, palpitations and breathlessness. Quickly determine if the situation is an emergency; does the patient need immediate resuscitation? Enquire about symptoms, examine the patient, and review the observations and drug and fluid-balance charts. Conduct some simple investigations to help determine if management with transfusion is required and tailor this to your specific patient.

HISTORY

Current medical problem

Why is the patient in hospital? Have they had a surgical procedure recently? Did they collapse in the community? Are they elderly? Ask whether there has been recent obvious bleeding such as haemoptysis, haematemesis, melaena, haematuria, epistaxis or heavy vaginal bleeding.

Current fluid status

Consider the patient's fluid intake, output and causes of extra fluid losses: do they balance out?

Intake

Has their medical/surgical condition stopped them from drinking enough water? If so, have they had enough replacement for their age and size? Assess the quantity of input from the following:

1. Oral intake – All types of fluid
2. Intravenous fluids (IVFs) – Note types of fluids (crystalloids, colloids, blood) and electrolyte composition
3. Parenteral feeding – Note electrolyte composition
4. Enteral feeding via nasogastric tubes (NGT), nasojejunal tubes and percutaneous endoscopic gastrostomies (PEGs)

Output

Assess all routes of output and insensible losses a patient might have. It is especially important to assess whether there is ongoing blood loss; has the patient noted blood in their stool/urine/vomit/surgical drain/wound site?

Signs and symptoms of fluid depletion can be vague, but put in context with the fluid balance chart, they should support your diagnosis. It is important to look at trends, as they will reveal the cause of fluid abnormality. For example, a patient may become progressively hypotensive due to ongoing blood loss and the observation chart will show a steady decline in blood pressure (BP), a rise in heart rate (HR) and altered respiratory rate (RR).

Hypovolaemia

- **Symptoms:** Thirst, oliguria/anuria, orthostatic hypotension, headache, lethargy, confusion, vomiting, diarrhoea.
- **Signs:** Decreased skin turgor, increased capillary refill time (CRT), cool peripheries, dry mucous membranes, tachycardia, weak thready pulse, tachypnoea, hypotension, increased RR, coma. These signs may not respond to fluid challenge, giving a clue to acute blood loss.

Table 6.1   Signs and symptoms of hypovolaemia by fluid compartment

Compartment	Symptoms of hypovolaemia	Signs of hypovolaemia
Intravascular	*Thirst, nausea*	*Tachycardia, hypotension*
Interstitial	*Thirst, nausea*	*No oedema, dry mucous membranes, poor skin turgor*

Think about the different fluid compartments. Table 6.1 presents the signs and symptoms of hypovolaemia associated with each compartment.

Past medical history

A patient's history will guide blood component prescribing. Have they previously received blood transfusions? If so, which components and was there a reaction? They may now have antibodies that might mean obtaining compatible blood takes a longer time. Your history should outline conditions that could affect current fluid status and highlight any indications for cautious prescribing. Focus on the following:

- **Haematological** – Presence of haemoglobinopathies such as sickle cell disease, haemolytic diseases and clotting factor disorders such as haemophilia. Also ask about a known vascular malformation, which could predispose to bleeding.

    - Most patients with β-thalassaemia major require red cell transfusions every 4 weeks or so to maintain their HbA levels above 95 g/L; anaemia can occur if the patient's schedule of transfusion is not individualised. Sickle cell disease patients have chronic anaemia and require red cell transfusion in acute crises and to prevent long-term organ damage when HbS fractions rise.

    - Consider undiagnosed haemophilia or von Willebrand disease if there is a personal or family history of unprovoked bleeding; the patient will need tests for these conditions and recombinant activated factor VII, VIII or desmopressin (releases factor VIIIc and von Willebrand factor [vWF] from endothelial cells to treat or prevent bleeding).

- **Hypoalbuminaemia** – Associated with inflammatory conditions, liver failure, nephrotic syndrome, malignancy and chronic illness. Hypoalbuminaemia reduces colloid osmotic pressure, contributing to oedema. This also inhibits platelet aggregation, therefore inhibiting clotting and cessation of blood loss. Distribution and metabolism of protein-bound drugs such as warfarin is altered in hypoalbuminaemia, increasing the risk of overcoagulation and bleeding.

- **Cardiovascular** – Ischaemic heart disease (IHD) and HF will affect the heart's ability to pump blood around the body in varying degrees. There may be pre-existing fluid overload. Be cautious when prescribing blood, as decreased cardiac output might result in excess fluid outside the intravascular space (oedema).

- **Renal** – Depending on the extent and cause of acute kidney injury (AKI) a patient may require careful transfusion, or dialysis first. Chronic kidney disease (CKD) of varying degrees will affect how the body processes external fluids and blood, and hence, the quantity and rate at which blood components are administered may need to be reduced. Ask if the patient is receiving erythropoietin, which increases the rate of production of red blood cells (RBCs), thus helping to prevent anaemia.

Medication

Take particular note of medications that affect the function of coagulation, the heart, kidneys and hormonal control of fluid and electrolyte balance. Some of these medications may need to be omitted or optimised before elective surgery or during an emergency admission; consult the *British National Formulary* (BNF), a clinical pharmacology text or a senior if you are unsure. The following are common medications in the general population and the effects that will influence your management:

- **Anticoagulants** – e.g. warfarin, dabigatran, rivaroxaban, heparin. Concurrent illness/incorrect dosing/drug interaction/surgery can lead to bleeding which is difficult to control. Reversing the anticoagulant effect can be tricky and lead to long-term problems re-establishing anticoagulation.

- **Antiplatelet drugs/nonsteroidal anti-inflammatory drugs (NSAIDs)** – e.g. aspirin, ibuprofen, clopidogrel, prasugrel. Aspirin and clopidogrel irreversibly impair platelet activation and cross-linking, an effect that can take up to 7 days to stop. NSAIDs have a shorter half-life and a reversible effect on prostaglandin synthesis. These drugs can lead to bleeding, especially if there is an interaction with cytochrome P450 (CYP450) inhibitors.

- **Antifibrinolytics** – e.g. tranexamic acid. To help control acute bleeding, especially in massive haemorrhage, menorrhagia, epistaxis and haemophilia. Can also be used in bleeding caused by over anticoagulation.

- **Steroids** – Used for a variety of conditions, can lead to side effects, which are more likely in higher doses. These include peptic/oeseophageal ulcers, thromboembolism, congestive cardiac failure (CCF) and generalised fluid and electrolyte imbalances.
- **Potassium sparing diuretics** – e.g. spironolactone can cause hyperkalaemia, hyponatraemia and water depletion. Stored red cells release potassium which could contribute to existing hyperkalaemia.
- **Electrolyte supplements** – e.g. potassium supplements will increase serum potassium levels; consider stopping them if red cell transfusion is required.
- **ACE inhibitors** – Renal impairment, increasing the risk of fluid overload with transfusions.
- **Beta-blockers** – Can cause decreased cardiac output, which will affect tissue perfusion in the event of hypovolaemia secondary to bleeding.
- **Furosemide** – Loop diuretic which can be used to offload excess fluid in frail patients or those with HF. This is administered in between blood transfusions to help avoid volume overload.

REMEMBER

Warfarin

In acute bleeding, especially if international normalised ratio (INR) >1.5, stop warfarin, give 5 mg vitamin K intravenously and 25–50 IU/kg of four-factor prothrombin complex concentrate (e.g. Beriplex, Octaplex). Pre-operatively, stop warfarin 5 days beforehand, replace with low-molecular-weight heparin up to 24 hours before the procedure if high risk of thrombosis.

Direct thrombin inhibitors (Dabigatran) and direct factor Xa inhibitors (Rivaroxaban, Apixaban)

These newer oral anticoagulants also have the side effect of haemorrhage, but less so than with warfarin. No current antidotes, but relatively short half-life of 5–20 hours depending on renal function. Tranexamic acid and haemodialysis may help; seek haematology advice.

Heparin

Unfractionated heparin may be used to treat and prevent venous thrombosis, but has the side effects of haemorrhage and thrombocytopaenia. The half-life of a continuous infusion is dependent on the dose and presence of renal impairment, varying from around 30 to 150 minutes. Therapeutic dosing requires 4–6 hourly clotting samples to determine the activated partial thromboplastin time (APTT) ratio (comparison of the APTT of the patient with that of normal pooled plasma). Stopping the infusion is usually sufficient to treat overdose, but rarely, reversal with protamine (protein that binds heparin, 1 mg for 100 IU heparin, maximum 50 mg) may be required.

Low-molecular-weight heparins, e.g. Enoxaparin, Tinzaparin, also treat and prevent venous thrombosis with the advantage of easier use, reduced need for monitoring and less effects on platelets. Since they have a longer half-life than the unfractionated form, stop prophylactic doses 12 hours before surgery and treatment doses 24 hours before. Protamine has less potency in reducing anticoagulant effects in the event of haemorrhage.

Examination

Look for clues that suggest trauma, ongoing bleeding or decompensation from chronic anaemia. Are there signs of worsening HF, for instance, and is there a new-onset arrhythmia? Assess the abdomen; is it tense, tender and becoming more distended over a short period of time (intra-abdominal bleeding)?

Use the 'ABCDE' approach to assess and manage the patient who has signs of hypovolaemic shock (see Chapter 3).

Late signs of bleeding such as bruising to the surrounding skin, flank (Grey Turner's sign) or peri-umbilicus (Cullen's sign) may be present. Signs of chronic anaemia include skin and conjunctival pallor, cheilosis, angular stomatitis, koilonychia and jaundice (see Figure 6.1).

Examine the orifices for clues about the source of bleeding, and inspect recent venepuncture/cannula/central line sites for bleeding; this could indicate disseminated intravascular coagulation (DIC). Also focus on the following signs outlined in Table 6.2.

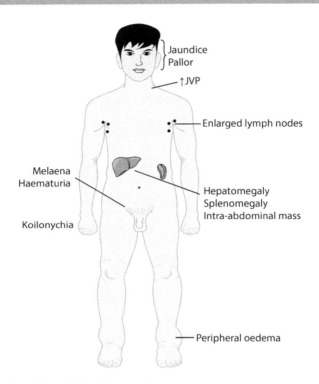

Figure 6.1   Signs of chronic anaemia.

Table 6.2   Signs of fluid depletion in ongoing bleeding

System	Fluid depletion
Cardiovascular	• Tachycardia? • Hypotension? • Capillary refill time (CRT) >2 seconds? • Decreased skin turgor? • Dry mucous membranes? • Postural drop in blood pressure?
Respiratory	• Respiratory rate (RR) >20 breaths/min?
Renal	• Decreased urine output <0.5 mL/kg/hr? • Concentrated urine?
Neurological	• Low Glasgow Coma Scale (GCS) <8? • Comatose? Meningism? Retinal signs? (may be associated with CNS bleed)

Most importantly, talk to the patient; determine if their airway is patent. Is their breathing pattern altered? Do they remain coherent or are they acutely confused, as can occur in haemorrhagic shock? You may need to abandon a full examination if you find abnormalities that require immediate resuscitation and additional help.

Investigations

By arranging the appropriate investigations, you play a crucial role in determining the cause of anaemia/bleeding, stopping bleeding, determining whether the patient requires a transfusion or other intervention and if so, ensuring that this is conducted safely. As you are not expected to request highly specialised tests when investigating anaemia, we will focus on the more common tests you will be expected to request and understand (see Table 6.3).

1. **Blood tests:** Especially important are an up-to-date measurement of the patient's full blood count (FBC), urea, electrolyte, liver function and clotting screen results. A blood film gives more information if aspects of the FBC result are abnormal. A Hemocue test gives a quick estimation of Hb level, as does an arterial blood gas (ABG), which may also show low oxygen saturation and mixed acidosis in haemorrhage. For instance, a patient with ongoing haemolysis may have a rising trend in unconjugated bilirubin. DIC would prolong APTT, raise INR and deplete platelet counts.

   Clotting Screen Helps monitor effect of interventions such as anticoagulants. Useful in those at risk of developing DIC, e.g. massive haemorrhage, severe sepsis, burns. Consider repeated clotting screens in bleeding that is difficult to control (is DIC developing?). Screening for DIC consists of checking prothrombin time (PT), APTT, fibrinogen, fibrin split products, and platelet count. This is confirmed by elevated coagulation times, decreased platelet counts and fibrinogen, and the presence of fibrin split products (see Table 6.4).

   Group and Save (G&S) samples should be collected, labelled by the bedside and checked with another health care professional to avoid transfusion errors. Laboratories analyse for ABO and rhesus D (RhD) grouping as well as common red cell antibodies. This information is stored so that specific blood components compatible with the patient can be prepared within 45 minutes of a subsequent request.

Table 6.3 Full blood count

Parameter	Interpretation
Haemoglobin	↔ or ↓ as anaemia advances.
Red blood cell (RBC) count	↓ in anaemia, haemolysis, massive transfusion. ↑ to compensate for low oxygen levels, in plasma fluid loss and bone marrow dysfunction.
Reticulocyte count	↑ in acute or chronic blood loss, haemolytic anaemia. ↓ in iron, B_{12} or folate deficiency, bone marrow failure, aplastic anaemia.
White blood cell (WBC) count	↑ in infection, inflammation, cancer. ↓ in bone marrow failure, severe infections.
Haematocrit/packed cell volume (PCV)	Same findings as RBC count.
Mean corpuscular volume (MCV)	↑ in B_{12} or folate deficiency, liver disease. ↓ in iron deficiency, thalassaemia, chronic disease.
Mean corpuscular haemoglobin (MCH)	May ↓ in iron deficiency, thalassaemia, inflammation.
Mean corpuscular haemoglobin concentration (MCHC)	As in the previous row.
Red cell distribution width (RDW)	↑ due to variation in size and shape of RBCs in some forms of anaemia, e.g. iron or B_{12} deficiency.
Platelets	↑ in inflammation, bleeding, iron deficiency, splenectomy, cancer. ↓ in disseminated intravascular coagulation (DIC), chronic bleeding, aplastic anaemia, Idiopathic Thrombocytopenic Purpura (ITP), splenomegaly, liver disease, many other causes.
Mean platelet volume	↑ when larger, younger, more reactive platelets are present, indicates high platelet destruction and turnover. ↓ in impaired production of platelets.

Crossmatch differs in that the patient's information is paired with a compatible stored blood component, a quicker process. This may be required in advance of a procedure if the patient has atypical antibodies and is at risk of requiring a transfusion.

Liver function and electrolyte tests In liver dysfunction, synthesis of proteins such as clotting factors is affected, leading to raised PT, and low albumin levels. Aspartate aminotransferase (AST) and alanine aminotransferase (ALT) levels increase in hepatocellular damage. Bilirubin level is raised in high rates of destruction of RBCs as occurs in haemolytic anaemia and sickle cell crises. Urea elevated more than creatinine suggests bleeding from the gastrointestinal tract. Electrolyte disturbance can exacerbate abnormal fluid shift patterns in anaemia. Transfusion can lead to hypocalcaemia and hyperkalaemia; therefore serial tests of electrolyte levels should be used as a baseline and to monitor for these side effects when managing bleeding.

Additional blood tests that may be helpful in evaluating anaemia include the following:

a. Haemoglobinopathy screen to help determine if a previously undiagnosed haemoglobinopathy such as sickle cell disease or β-thalassaemia is the cause of anaemia
b. Iron studies
c. Folate and B_{12} levels
d. Blood film
e. Coombs test
f. Clotting factor assay (factors II, V, VII, IX, X, XI, XII) and Protein C and S levels
g. Antibody screening, e.g. to intrinsic factor in B_{12} deficiency
h. Virology tests, e.g. cytomegalovirus (CMV), Epstein–Barr virus (EBV)
i. Bone marrow aspiration
j. Toxicology screening

Table 6.4 Clotting screen results in coagulation disorders

Disorder	INR	APTT	Prothrombin time (PT)	Platelet count	Bleeding time
Disseminated intravascular coagulation (DIC)	↑↑	↑↑	↑↑	↓	↑
Von Willebrand's	↔	↑↑	↔	↔	↑
Haemophilia	↔	↑↑	↔	↔	↔
Platelet defect	↔	↔	↔	↔	↑
Liver disease	↑	↑	↔/↑	↔/↓	↔/↑
Heparin	↑	↑↑	↑↑	↔	↔
Vitamin K deficiency	↑↑	↑	↑	↔	↔

2. **Urine:** Gross haematuria warrants further assessment of the renal function/tract for stones, malignancy, benign prostatic hyperplasia or obstruction. Microscopic urinalysis may confirm the presence of RBCs/casts, seen in tubular or glomerular causes of bleeding; urine cytology provides more information. Albuminuria suggests renal impairment, especially if the albumin–creatinine ratio is also raised. Elevated urobilinogen/haemosiderin levels may indicate haemolysis.

3. **Electrocardiogram:** Essential for assessment of any current cardiac ischaemia or rhythm abnormality secondary to bleeding – blood component and fluid therapy will depend on the extent and cause of the problem. Where possible, look at previous ECGs and compare for any signs of atrial fibrillation, myocardial infarction or dysrhythmias.

4. **Imaging:** Useful to help determine if there is abnormal fluid distribution, such as chest x-ray (CXR) findings in pulmonary oedema. Furthermore, imaging allows investigation into the clinical cause of abnormal fluid distribution, such as transfusion-associated circulatory overload, or a cardiac or renal abnormality.

   a. Radiographs – CXR for any signs of fluid overload, haemothorax

   b. Echocardiogram – Left ventricular ejection fraction (LVEF), ventricular enlargement, dysfunctional pumping

   c. Ultrasound scan – Ruptured abdominal aortic aneurysm (AAA), intra-abdominal or wound-site haematomas, splenic rupture, renal hydronephrosis

   d. Computed tomography (CT) – CT of the head for intra-cranial bleed or of the abdomen for suspected leaking AAA, intra-abdominal collections. CT cystourethrogram in suspected bladder trauma/malignancy

BLOOD COMPONENTS

Following rigorous screening, donor blood is processed into blood components such as red cell and platelet concentrates, fresh frozen plasma (FFP) and cryoprecipitate. Plasma from donor blood is processed and incorporated into blood plasma derivatives such as factors VIII and X, human albumin solution and immunoglobulins (Figure 6.2).

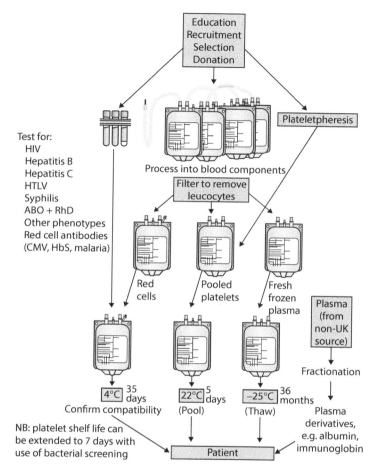

Figure 6.2 Production of blood components and blood derivatives. (From Derek N, *Handbook of Transfusion Medicine*, Norwich, UK: United Kingdom Blood Services, 2013. With permission.)

Whole blood

A unit of whole blood consists of around 405–495 mL of leucocyte-depleted blood with added citrate phosphate dextrose anticoagulant. This is no longer commonly used in the United Kingdom, due to the unnecessary risk of reactions to components of blood transfused. This maximises the ways in which donor blood can be split into different components and used to help as many people as possible.

Red cells

Indication: To restore oxygen-carrying capacity in severe anaemia or ongoing bleeding, where alternative treatments are ineffective or not appropriate.

Practical points: Plasma is removed from donated blood and replaced with an additive solution. A typical unit has a volume of 220–340 mL, raises Hb levels by around 10 g/L and can be stored for up to 35 days. Stored at 2°C–6°C, it must be started within 30 minutes of removal from the blood fridge and completed within 4 hours. Low viscosity allows a red cell unit to be squeezed in where necessary. Ideally, it should be crossmatched to a recent sample from the patient to avoid ABO incompatibility; in an emergency O RhD-negative blood can be used.

Irradiated red cells are used for patients at risk of transfusion-associated graft-versus-host disease, e.g. organ transplant patients on specific immunosuppressors. Gamma or x-rays are used within 14 days of receiving donated blood and the product must then be used within 14 days.

Washed red cells are used for patients with recurrent, severe allergic or febrile reactions and IgA-deficient patients with anti-IgA antibodies. Preparation involves removal of all but traces of plasma.

REMEMBER

Normal Hb values:
Men: 130–180 g/L   Women: 110–150 g/L
Consider blood transfusion if the Hb is between/or <70–80 g/L **and** the patient is symptomatic. Quickly decide upon and arrange transfusion of red cells in case of massive haemorrhage. Assess your implemented treatment and decide whether further amounts or types of blood components are required.

A unit of red cells gives an increment of around 10 g/L, but this applies to a standard weight of 70–80 kg. The number of units prescribed should be less if the patient weighs less than this, to avoid fluid overload.

A transfused volume of 4 mL/kg will generally give an increment of 10 g/L. Low-weight adults and all children should have their transfusion prescribed in millilitres rather than units to avoid potential overload.

Platelets

Indication: Treatment or prevention of bleeding in those with thrombocytopaenia or platelet dysfunction (could be secondary to massive haemorrhage).

Practical points: 200–300 mL/unit. Stored at 20°C–24°C for 5–7 days, must be kept agitated. Adult therapeutic dose is >240 × 10⁹/unit. Platelet transfusions should be selected to be compatible with a patient's blood group, as platelets have ABO antigens on their surface. Produced in two ways; the majority by apheresis from a single donor or by pooling from four donors.

Irradiated platelets are used for the same indications as the irradiated red cells mentioned previously.

Platelets in additive solution are obtained by washing to remove plasma. Only available for use for 24 hours after this process. Used in those who have previously had severe allergic or febrile reactions to standard platelet transfusions.

Human leukocyte antigen (HLA)-selected platelets are used in those with HLA antibodies developed after previous transfusions. **Human platelet antigens (HPAs)-selected platelets** are used for babies with neonatal alloimmune thrombocytopaenia.

Fresh frozen plasma

Indication: Treatment of patients with bleeding in the presence of single or multiple clotting factor deficiency. No longer indicated for warfarin reversal; use prothrombin complex instead if required. Do not use as a plasma volume expander as there is the risk of a severe allergic reaction.

Practical points: Obtained from male donors only (reduces risk of transfusion-related acute lung injury [TRALI]). Around 250 mL/unit, adult dose requires at least 4 units, as amount of individual clotting factors per unit varies. Stored for up to 36 months at –25°C or below. Use immediately or within 24 hours of thawing if stored at 4°C. Use immediately or within 4 hours of thawing if stored at room temperature.

FFP can be processed via a solvent detergent pooling method to further inactivate microbes (including HIV) and standardise the levels of clotting factors in each pack. Methylene blue treatment of single donor FFP also further inactivates microbes and is preferred in some paediatric settings.

Cryoprecipitate

Indication: Initially developed for haemophilia treatment (factor VIII concentrate used instead nowadays), now mainly used as a more concentrated, lower infused volume source of fibrinogen than FFP.

Practical points: Made by thawing FFP at 4°C to produce a cryoglobulin rich in fibrinogen, factor VIII and vWF. Can also be produced from methylene blue processed FFP. Single donor pack (average 43 mL) or pool from five donors (average 189 mL). Stored for up to 36 months at −25°C or below. Use immediately or within 4 hours of thawing, cannot be re-refrigerated.

Granulocytes

Indication: Used in those with severe neutropenia with life-threatening bacterial or fungal infection. More commonly used in those with severe neutropenia after cytotoxic chemotherapy or bone marrow failure.

Practical points: Prepared from whole blood as buffy coats or by apheresis from individual donors. Irradiated before use and must be group compatible with the recipient. Must be approved by a senior haematologist. Stored at 20°C–24°C, should not be agitated. Stored for 24 hours only and should be administered over 1–2 hours. Daily infusions may be given until evidence of recovery occurs, if there is decline despite several consecutive transfusions or if a severe reaction occurs.

Individual buffy coats contain red cells and platelets in addition to granulocytes, reducing the need for concurrent platelet and red cell transfusions. Around 10 packs of 60 mL each are required to achieve a daily dose, 10–20 mL/kg in those weighing less than 30 kg.

Pooled buffy coats have lower volumes and less red cell and plasma content, with a reduced need for platelet and red cell transfusions. 10 donations are pooled into a pack volume of 200–250 mL with platelet additive solution. Two packs are required for a standard adult dose, 10–20 mL/kg in those weighing less than 30 kg.

Apheresis granulocytes are obtained from relatives or friends who are HLA-compatible with the recipient. These samples contain much higher numbers of granulocytes, as the donors receive granulocyte colony stimulating factor and steroids before sample collection.

A patient may require more than one type of blood product. This decision depends on the patient's symptoms, estimated amount of blood lost and the mechanism through which this has happened; see the section on 'Transfusion regimes' for more on this.

BLOOD PRODUCTS

The term blood products describes blood plasma derivatives manufactured from pooled plasma donations from countries with low risk of variant Creutzfeldt–Jakob disease. All products are subject to pathogen-inactivation processing steps to remove transfusion-transmitted viruses and other microbes.

Human albumin solution

Indication: Isotonic solution (3.5%–5.5%) used in acute or subacute loss of plasma volume as seen in burns and pancreatitis for example. Also used as a replacement fluid in plasma exchange therapy. Concentrated solution (20%) used in severe hypoalbuminaemia with low plasma volume and generalised oedema, e.g. in cirrhosis or nephrotic syndrome; aims to expand plasma volume despite salt and fluid intake restriction. Also used when large volumes of ascites are drained in patients with portal hypertension for example.

Practical points: Contains no blood group antibodies or clotting factors. Available in 50-mL, 100-mL or 500-mL preparations. Administer slowly in those with circulatory failure to avoid further overload. Prescribed as a medicinal product; see your local or national formulary for prescription details.

Clotting factor concentrates

Indication: Treatment or prophylaxis of bleeding in those with congenital or acquired coagulation disorders. Single factor concentrates are available for most congenital deficiencies, except for deficiencies of factors II and V. Discuss the appropriate choice of concentrate with a local senior haematologist on-call before prescribing or ordering.

Recombinant factor VIIIc is used in Haemophilia A, while **recombinant factor IX** is used in Haemophilia B. **Dried factor VIII fraction** contains varying amounts of vWF, and is used where a bleeding episode is not improved by desmopressin. It may also contain factors II, VII and X.

Recombinant factor VIIa (NovoSeven) is used in factor VII deficiency, haemophilia with inhibitors to factor VIII and IX and acquired haemophilia. It is also used in intracranial haemorrhage and diffuse alveolar haemorrhage and can be given in boluses during an acute bleeding episode.

Fibrinogen concentrate (factor I) is used in congenital or acquired (DIC, massive transfusion) hypofibrinogenaemia. **Dried factor XIII**

fraction (human fibrin-stabilising factor) is used in congenital factor XIII deficiency.

Prothrombin complex concentrate (e.g. Beriplex, Octaplex) contains factors II, VII, IX and X. Now used instead of FFP to reverse warfarin overdose in active or expected bleeding, at a dose of 25–50 IU/kg, under haematology guidance. Also used to treat coagulopathy secondary to liver disease.

Immunoglobulin solutions

Normal immunoglobulin is manufactured from normal plasma and contains antibodies to viruses such as hepatitis A, rubella and measles. It is given in intramuscular doses to those who may be susceptible to infection with these viruses. In high intravenous doses, normal immunoglobulin is used as a replacement in severe immunoglobulin deficiency and in autoimmune conditions such as idiopathic thrombocytopenic purpura (ITP). Normal immunoglobulin is contraindicated in those with IgA deficiency with a known IgA antibody because of the risk of life-threatening allergic reaction or anaphylaxis mediated by possible IgG anti-IgA antibodies.

Specific immunoglobulins are obtained from selected donors with high plasma levels of antibodies to tetanus, hepatitis B, rabies, varicella zoster and anti-D for example.

TRANSFUSION REGIMES

After a thorough clinical assessment, a decision should be made about whether the transfusion of one or more blood components/products is appropriate, ensuring that the benefits outweigh the risk of harm. A recent crossmatch or G&S sample (some laboratories require a sample obtained within the previous 72 hours) should be used to prepare the right blood for the right patient.

Document the reason for transfusion, treatment target and the patient's consent in the clinical notes. Prescribe each unit to be administered and the duration of each unit; remember that in haemorrhage causing compromise, units should be administered 'stat' (over 5–10 minutes). Ensure that the patient has a working large bore peripheral cannula (at least green 18 gauge, with a flow rate of approximately 2.8 L/hr) or central venous catheter. IVF should not be given through the same infusion line as blood components, but through a different line or lumen of a multi-lumen catheter. Calcium in, e.g. Gelofusin and Hartmann's solution antagonises the citrate anticoagulant in blood components and rarely, may allow clots to form if administered in the same infusion line.

The term 'goal-directed therapy' in relation to blood transfusions refers to the need to ensure that patients only receive the type and number of blood components/products that they require and avoid over-transfusion and associated adverse effects. Therapy should be restrictive rather than liberal. What is the target Hb level? How many units of red cells will be necessary to achieve this?

Remember that in rapid acute blood loss, the Hb level does not drop immediately. This only occurs with dilution over time as the body shifts fluid between compartments to compensate, or as IVF is administered. Think of a bucket of blood; part of this is emptied, the overall volume of blood in the bucket is reduced, but the concentration remains the same.

Major haemorrhage

Major haemorrhage protocol exists in hospitals to co-ordinate the response to a significant loss of blood volume, as can be seen in trauma or surgical patients. Apart from clinicians, the haematology laboratory and porters are alerted so that blood components can be prepared and transported to the patient without delay. Major haemorrhage may be identified when bleeding leads to signs of haemorrhagic shock (systolic BP <90 mmHg, HR >100 bpm etc.); the patient is likely to have lost 30%–40% of circulating blood volume by this stage. Major haemorrhage may also be defined as blood loss of more than 150 mL/min, or 50% of blood volume loss within 3 hours or more than one blood volume loss within 24 hours (>70 mL/kg).

Aim to site two large bore cannulas, taking samples for FBC, clotting profile, fibrinogen, U+Es, LFTs and G&S. Whilst waiting for blood to arrive, replace intravascular fluid volume with a warmed, balanced crystalloid (Hartmann's, Plasmalyte) or colloid (Volpex, Gelofusin) if profound hypotension occurs. Do not hesitate to administer O RhD-negative blood if there is ongoing bleeding whilst waiting for group-specific blood. Tranexamic acid as a bolus or infusion is also useful in limiting fibrinolysis in major haemorrhage.

Major haemorrhage protocol often consists of two or more packs of blood components in differing amounts. An example is set out below, check your local hospital guideline to determine what your protocol consists of.

- **Pack 1** – 4 units of RBCs
- **Pack 2** – 6 units of RBCs, 4 units of FFP, 1 pool of platelets. 2 pools of cryoprecipitate if fibrinogen level <1.5 g/L

Pack 1 is issued in the first wave and then pack 2 and subsequent repeats of pack 2 are issued following assessment of the patient's response, whether there is ongoing bleeding and upon advice from a senior haematologist. In some cases of major haemorrhage, massive transfusion and coagulopathy, transfusion of RBC, FFP and platelet units is advocated in a near 1:1:1 approach. This is because transfusion of large volumes of IVF and RBCs leads to dilutional coagulopathy; platelet, fibrinogen and other clotting factor levels fall, especially when insufficient levels of platelets or FFP are transfused. Consumptive coagulopathy occurs when platelets and clotting factors are used up in the physiological response to trauma. Increased fibrinolysis, hypothermia, hypoxia, acidosis and hypocalcaemia also contribute to coagulopathy in major haemorrhage.

Massive transfusion can lead to metabolic disturbances such as hypocalcaemia. The citrate anticoagulant in blood components can bind to ionised calcium, which can lead to clinical manifestations of hypocalcaemia (treat with calcium chloride or gluconate as necessary).

REMEMBER

Standard administration of 2 units of red blood cells over 2–3 hours each.

In elderly patients or those with existing circulatory compromise such as heart failure, administer Furosemide 20–40-mg orally or intravenously after the second unit of red cells and then with each alternate unit thereafter.

Re-assess the patient within 2 hours of the initial transfusion. Has there been an adequate haemodynamic response? Have BP and HR returned to normal range? Urine output maintained at ≥0.5 mL/kg/hr?

Is there a need for further units of red blood cells? Are FFP, platelets or cryoprecipitate now indicated if there is ongoing bleeding or abnormal coagulation?

Consider instigating the major haemorrhage protocol if there is rapid ongoing blood loss or haemorrhagic shock develops.

As a minimum, monitoring of the patient receiving a blood transfusion should include temperature, pulse, BP and RR, with a baseline 0 minutes before the transfusion starts and then 15 minutes after this. Check these observations again within 60 minutes of completing each individual unit. If any symptoms of a reaction occur, check these observations again; if there is a significant change, consider stopping the transfusion and taking further action to stabilise the patient.

REVIEW THE IMPLEMENTED TREATMENT

REMEMBER

In patients who are actively bleeding, the platelet count should be maintained >50 × 10⁹/L, PT ratio >1.5 and fibrinogen >1.5 g/L. Hb level should be >70 g/L and >90 g/L in those with existing cardiovascular disease.

You must monitor the patient closely for warning signs of fluid overload, dehydration, electrolyte abnormalities (hypocalcaemia, hyperkalaemia), altered consciousness or other adverse outcome.

Complications of blood transfusions include immunological causes such as blood group incompatibility, haemolysis, graft-versus-host disease, transfusion-associated lung injury and urticaria. Non-immunological causes include transmission of infection, iron overload, electrolyte changes in massive transfusion and air embolism. Specifically, this text focuses on the identification and management of transfusion-associated circulatory overload.

Transfusion reaction screen

A reaction to the transfusion of blood products is classed as any that occurs within 24 hours of administration. Use the 'ABCDE' approach to assess and manage the patient, with the addition of adrenaline, hydrocortisone, chlorphenamine and IVFs if severe anaphylaxis occurs.

Screening investigations should include the following:

- Baseline FBC, renal and liver function, urinalysis.
- G&S sample for repeat compatibility and antibody testing.
- Return the blood component to the lab for bacterial contamination and compatibility testing.

- Mast cell tryptase levels rise after a true severe anaphylactic reaction; levels should be checked as soon as possible after the event and then at 3 and 24 hours after. Most useful where symptoms of anaphylaxis may be masked, such as under anaesthesia.

Transfusion associated circulatory overload

Transfusion associated circulatory overload (TACO) is acute or worsening pulmonary oedema within 6 hours of a blood transfusion. This is more common with RBC transfusions or transfusion of large volumes of blood components.

Features include tachycardia, hypertension, acute respiratory distress and positive fluid balance. Treatment involves stopping the transfusion and supportive management to move fluid from the pulmonary interstitium; oxygen, diuretics, close monitoring perhaps on a high dependency unit. The risk of TACO is reduced by careful clinical assessment before transfusion and calculating volumes to be transfused according to weight and in millilitres, not unit size. Close monitoring during transfusion can also help to identify TACO early.

CONCLUSION

Anaemia can be a life-threatening condition, especially if caused by acute haemorrhage. In assessing a patient for signs of acute anaemia or ongoing haemorrhage, take a detailed history, examine and conduct appropriate investigations. If there are signs of ongoing bleeding, address this quickly, instigating the local major haemorrhage protocol if necessary. Whole blood is no longer used to replace lost blood volume; different components such as RBCs, FFP and cryoprecipitate are used instead. This is done as 'goal-directed therapy', i.e. to maintain target Hb, PT, fibrinogen and platelet levels and avoid complications such as circulatory overload and metabolic disturbances. Blood products such as clotting factor concentrates and immunoglobulins are useful in managing congenital or acquired clotting disorders and immune-mediated conditions. Remember that senior members of your clinical team and haematologists are available for advice when managing patients who require blood components or blood products.

CASE 6.1 – UPPER GASTROINTESTINAL BLEED

A 57-year-old man with known heavy alcohol intake and tobacco abuse presents to hospital complaining of lethargy and foul-smelling black tarry stool. His observations are as follows:

HR 120 bpm
BP 80/40 mmHg
CRT 5 seconds
RR 22 breaths/min
O_2 saturation 88% on room air
Temperature 36°C

On examination, no stigmata of chronic liver disease are found. He has rhinophyma and epigastric tenderness on palpation; he admits to taking ibuprofen for the previous few days. During the consultation, he vomits around 100 mL of fresh blood and becomes confused.

What is the main abnormality and what is the most likely underlying diagnosis?

This man is displaying signs of hypovolaemic shock secondary to recent upper GI bleeding. He is tachycardic, hypotensive, hypoxic, hypothermic and has a narrow pulse pressure.

Hallmarks

- Melaena, epigastric pain and haematemesis are signs of upper GI bleeding.
- Peptic ulcer disease and oesophageal varices are the most common causes of upper GI bleeding.
- Hypovolaemic shock features severe hypotension, narrow pulse pressure, tachycardia and reduced tissue perfusion secondary to reduced intravascular fluid volume.

Management

- Call for help, move the patient to a bay in the resuscitation area of A&E.
- Use the 'ABCDE' approach to initiate resuscitation.
- Maintain his airway and oxygen saturation at 88%–92% (tobacco abuse and admission saturation of 88% suggests hypercapnic respiratory drive).
- Site two large bore cannulae and administer 500 mL of warm balanced crystalloid (Hartmann's or Plasmalyte) via a pressure bag.

CASE 6.1 (continued)

- High dose intravenous proton-pump inhibitor such as pantoprazole.
- Review ABG/venous blood gas (VBG) and FBC results, arrange blood transfusion as necessary, using the major haemorrhage protocol if fresh bleeding continues.
- Consider thiamine and alcohol withdrawal regimes once he is stable.

Investigations
- Hemocue or VBG to get a quick Hb result.
- FBC, G&S, clotting profile. U+Es.
- Erect CXR – looking for signs of perforation (peritoneal bleed).
- Arrange urgent endoscopy to determine if gastric/oesophageal ulcers are present and to stem ongoing bleeding.
- Consider urinary catheterisation to help monitor urine output i.e. end-organ perfusion.

CASE 6.2 – MASSIVE OBSTETRIC HAEMORRHAGE

Following a spontaneous vaginal delivery at home, a 24-year-old woman is transferred to labour ward via ambulance because the placenta has not delivered and she is estimated to have lost around 500 mL of fresh blood from the vagina so far. The paramedics have sited a 'green' cannula and an infusion of Hartmann's is running through. She is quickly transferred to the labour ward theatre for removal of the retained placenta.

Upon transfer from the bed to the theatre table, a large pool of blood is noted on the incontinence pad she has been lying on. This pad is subsequently weighed, adding another 250 mL to the total estimated blood volume lost. After the spinal anaesthetic and removal of the placenta, there is a sudden gush of blood from the vagina, the sterile drapes and incontinence pads on the floor are soaked.

She states that she feels faint and can no longer hear clearly. The anaesthetist also notes that she appears pale and her observations are as follows:

HR 125 bpm
BP 80/52 mmHg
CRT 5 seconds
RR 26 breaths/min
O_2 saturation 92% on room air
Temperature 37°C

What is the most likely underlying diagnosis?

Haemorrhagic shock in massive obstetric haemorrhage secondary to a retained placenta and uterine atony.

Hallmarks

- Massive obstetric haemorrhage can be brisk or rapidly accumulate over a short period of time.
- Young people cope with a large loss in circulating blood volume for longer than those who are frail or have an existing cardiopulmonary disease.
- Fibrinolysis can be more marked than in other causes of massive haemorrhage.
- Hypotension, tachycardia and hypoxia are features of haemorrhagic shock.

Management

- Use the 'ABCDE' approach to resuscitate the patient.
- Administer oxygen at 15 L/min via a non-rebreathe mask.
- Squeeze in 500 mL of a warm, balanced intravenous crystalloid through a pressure bag. Further fluid boluses may be required whilst awaiting blood.
- Estimate the total volume of blood lost, including weighing of the pads, drapes and blood clots. This will help decide whether the patient requires a certain number of RBC units only or a major haemorrhage protocol and therefore FFP, platelets and cryoprecipitate in addition.
- Aim to replace lost blood with transfused blood quickly; consider giving warmed O RhD-negative blood, which is kept in a fridge in most labour wards.
- Obstetric management includes bimanual uterine compression to help improve uterine tone, and pharmacological measures such as misoprostol, syntocinon and ergometrine.
- Continue the cycle of clinical and laboratory monitoring and administration of goal-directed blood component therapy until bleeding stops and the patient is stable.
- Seek senior obstetric and anaesthetic support with stabilising the patient. In some cases, patients need arterial and central venous lines and nursing in a high-dependency or intensive care setting so that they their response to treatment can be closely monitored and adjusted.

CASE 6.2 (continued)

Investigations

- Point-of-care testing such as Hemocue, ABG/VBG provide rapid information about the patient's current status.
- Laboratory samples of blood for FBC, clotting profile, fibrinogen, U+Es and G&S should be sent as soon as possible after admission, to provide baseline information.
- Further laboratory blood samples help guide ongoing management. For example, Hb count may be below target despite massive transfusion.
- If further vaginal bleeding occurs after the initial phase, pelvic ultrasound may be required to investigate for further retained products of conception.

Further reading

Birchall J, Stanworth SJ, Duffy MR, Doree CJ and Hyde C. Evidence for the use of recombinant factor VIIa in the prevention and treatment of bleeding in patients without haemophilia. *Transfus Med Rev* 2008; 22: 177–187.

British Committee for Standards in Haematology (BCSH). *Guideline on the Administration of Blood Components – Addendum on Avoidance of Transfusion Associated Circulatory Overload (TACO) and Problems Associated with Over-Transfusion*. 2012. http://www.bcshguidelines.com/documents/BCSH_Blood_Admin_-_addendum_August_2012.pdf.

British National Formulary. www.bnf.org.uk.

Derek N. *Handbook of Transfusion Medicine*, 5th Edition. Norwich, UK: United Kingdom Blood Services, 2013.

London Regional Transfusion Committee. *Care Pathways for the Management of Adult Patients Refusing Blood (Including Jehovah's Witnesses Patients)*. http://www.transfusionguidelines.org.uk/docs/pdfs/rtc-lo_2012_05_jw_policy.pdf.

Nathalie H, James D, Stephan S and Simon E. *Oxford Handbook for the Foundation Programme*, 2nd Edition. Oxford, UK: Oxford University Press, 2008.

Patrick D. *Medicine at a Glance*, 4th Edition. Chichester, UK: Wiley-Blackwell, June 2014.

Peck TE and Hill SA. Pharmacology for Anaesthesia and Intensive Care, 4th Edition. Cambridge, UK: Cambridge University Press, 2014.

Tinegate H, Birchall J, Gray A, et al. Guideline on the investigation and management of acute transfusion reactions. Prepared by the BCSH Blood Transfusion Task Force. *Br J Haematol* 2012; 159(2): 143–153.

Index